Contents

Author's Foreword

With the rapid development of Western medicine, medical costs have become an increasing burden to everyone. That is one reason more and more attention is being paid to natural therapies such as self-massage along meridians and acupoints. A traditional Chinese therapy with a successful cure rate that involves simple manipulation with no side effects, self-massage is popular in many countries: It is a proven rehabilitative method of strengthening the body to prevent and treat disease as well as to prolong life. Over years of study and practice, I have worked to improve this traditional therapy in ways that include collecting my experience in the field into this book, *Self-Massage Along Meridians and Acupoints.*

I was born in December 1934 into a peasant's family of the Gelo ethnic minority in Guizhou Province. My family has practiced self-massage along meridians and acupoints for three generations, although I am now the only one in the family to continue this tradition. I also have studied the literature on self-massage published in the Tang, Ming and Qing dynasties. In the past 40 years, I have treated over 400,000 patients to develop my own abilities in healing-skills characterized in China as "iron arm, water wrist and embroidery hand." I have published 20 articles and several monographs which have been translated into English, German, Russian, Malay, Czech, Portuguese and Spanish. They include *Practical Chinese Self-Massage Along Meridians and Acupoints, Chinese Family Self-Massage Along Meridians and Acupoints* and *Major Systems of Traditional Chinese Medicine: Clinical Massage Therapy for Basic Levels.* Some of my work is now available on videotape. I am listed in *China's "Who's Who" of Doctors* and the *World Dictionary of Notable Doctors (Chinese Volume).*

I now serve as director, chief physician and professor in the Rehabilitative Department of Physical Medicine in the Administrative Bureau Hospital attached to the Headquarters of the General Staff of the People's Liberation Army. I am a guest professor at the clinic of the Chinese Academy of Traditional Chinese Medicine, and a member of the Beijing Branch of the China Association of Integrated Chinese and Western Medicine. I am director of the Traumatology and Orthopedics Association; vice director of Traumatology-Orthopedics and Massage Association of the People's Liberation Army; and a member of the Beijing Bone-setting and Massage Association of Traditional Chinese Medicine.

My experience in massage therapy includes treating cervical vertebral disease, protrusion of lumbar vertebral disc, paralysis, diabetes, neurasthenia, rheumatic arthritis, impotence, irregular menstruation and menopause. Having witnessed the remarkable effects of traditional massage therapy, I began to develop my own system of self-massage along meridians and acupoints for strengthening the body, preventing diseases and general healthcare. I have visited many countries including the United States, France, Portugal, Romania, Pakistan, Jordan and Oman, where I was invited to treat army and government leaders.

Self-Massage Along Meridians and Acupoints, with its in-depth content and accompanying illustrations, is a good reference book both for general readers as well as for doctors and nurses of traditional Chinese medicine and Western medicine. In the 21st century, the mysteries of meridians and acupoints will become better understood, and as more and more patients benefit from this therapy — and other effective methods — the average life span of human beings will be 90 years or more. I will continue to devote myself to the study of self-massage along meridians and acupoints with the hope of continuing to improve this therapy in the advancement of traditional Chinese medicine.

Wang Chuangui
December 1998
Beijing

Chapter 1
General Introduction

Section 1 History of Self-Massage Along Meridians and Acupoints

Chinese therapeutic massage (*Tuina*) was used for medical purposes in China as early as the Spring and Autumn period, about 2,000 years ago. It says in the "Basic Questions" of the *Yellow Emperor's Classic of Internal Medicine*, the earliest extant medical canon published in the Warring States (475-221 BC): "Massage and decoction (a therapeutic tea made from herbs) can be used to treat numbness due to an obstruction of meridians created by repeated fright." This shows that in the ancient times massage was already a specialty and applied in clinical treatment along with decoction.

History also records in the section on "Official Positions" in the *New Tang Dynasty Book* that the imperial hospitals in the dynasties of Sui (581-618) and Tang (618-907) had one chief doctor responsible for massage and four massage therapists, ranked grade nine, responsible for the treatment of diseases and traumatic injury with massage and *daoyin* (physical movements executed in coordination with controlled breathing)."

The Six Canons of the Tang Dynasty reports that massage can be used to cure eight kinds of diseases, namely, diseases due to wind, cold, summer-heat, dampness, hunger, overeating, stress and inactivity.

In the dynasties of Song (960-1279), Kin (1115-1234) and Yuan (1271-1368), massage therapy was used extensively. According to the *General Collection of Prescriptions*: "Simultaneous application of pressing and rubbing is called massage while pressing without rubbing or rubbing without pressing is called pressing therapy or rubbing therapy which have their own specific indications."

In the Ming (1368-1644) and Qing (1644-1911) dynasties, massage therapy was developed further. During that period medicine was divided into 13 specialties, one of which was massage. Much experience was accumulated in the treatment of children's diseases, which brought about a specific system of pediatric massage.

With the founding of the People's Republic of China in 1949, massage therapy has developed remarkably in the modern era.

Section 2 The Definition of Self-Massage Along Meridians and Acupoints

Self-massage along meridians and acupoints is one of the unique traditional therapies developed in ancient China based on the theory of *qi* and blood as well as viscera and meridians. It is performed by rubbing the meridians, acupoints, 12 tendons and 12 divisions of skin with different parts of the hands. The techniques employed usually are kneading and holding the tendons as well as rubbing and stroking the skin for softening and lubricating the tendons and bones so as to cure diseases. Since this therapy is used to treat diseases by the patient himself or herself, it is called "self-massage along meridians and acupoints."

Section 3 Overview

1. Names of the Regions of the Body

To perform self-massage along meridians and acupoints, one has to have general knowledge about the skeleton and muscles, especially the names of their regions in the body, to be able to determine accurate location (Figs 1 and 2).

The body is divided into head, neck, trunk and four limbs.

The head is further divided into face, forehead, crown and occipital region.

The neck is divided into neck and nape.

The trunk is divided into chest, back, waist and abdomen [the abdomen is divided into upper abdomen, left hypochondrium (the upper lateral region of the abdomen, marked by the lower ribs), right hypochondrium, navel, pubic region, left groin and right groin].

The four limbs are divided into shoulder, upper arm, elbow, forearm, wrist, palm, buttock, hip, thigh, knee, shank, ankle and foot.

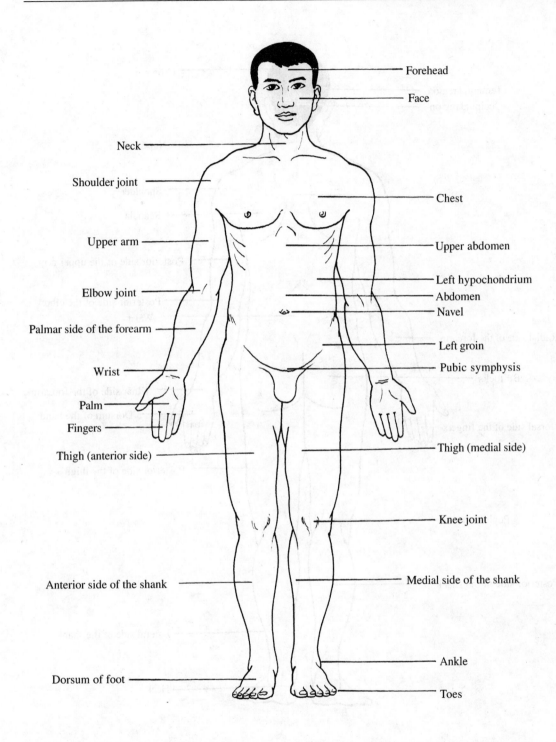

Fig. 1 Names of the main parts of the human body surface (front)

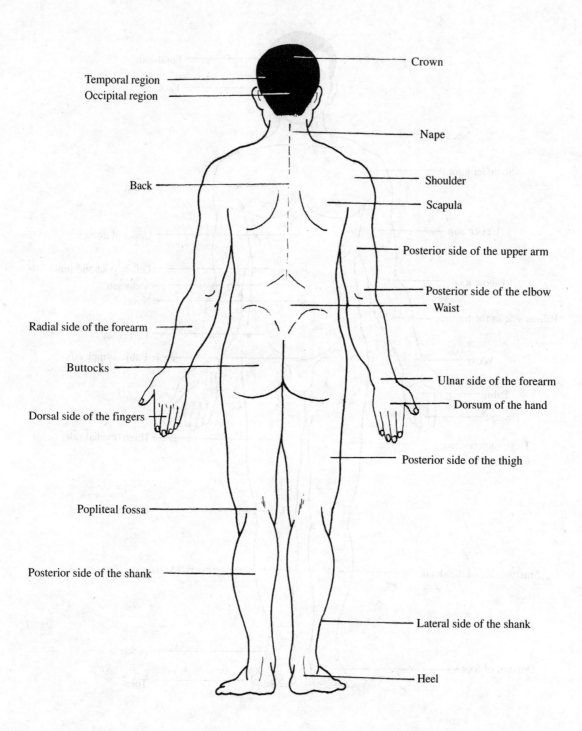

Fig. 2 Names of the main parts of the human body surface (back)

2. Essentials for Successful Self-Massage Along Meridians and Acupoints

(1) Accurate diagnosis is a must in the application of self-massage along meridians and acupoints.

(2) The area of the body to be massaged must be exposed, with the hand directly touching the body surface. To reduce resistance and to avoid damage to the skin, certain kinds of medicinal liquids, oils, wines and powders can be applied to the region prior to massage.

(3) Hand techniques must be swift, gentle, moderate and steady, according to the situation. The session starts from comfort to relaxed comfort. Frequent and regular self-massage along meridians and acupoints will achieve the best result.

(4) Each massage session should last for 20-30 minutes. Sensations that can be expected during massage are local aching, numbness and distention, which are normal, especially when the acupoints are pressed and rubbed to produce what is called "needling sensation."

(5) Massage should be avoided when one feels hungry. Massage should not be applied to the abdomen within one hour after meal. Urination and defecation should be done prior to application of massage to the abdomen.

3. Contraindication — When One Should Not Apply Self-Massage Along Meridians and Acupoints

(1) Infectious diseases and open wounds (including erysipelas, abscess, tuberculosis of bones and joints, osteomyelitis, phlegmon and suppurative arthritis, etc.)

(2) Hemorrhagic diseases (such as scurvy and malignant anemia)

(3) Various malignant tumors.

(4) Pregnancy. Women with lumbar and abdominal disorders should not be treated during pregnancy or menstruation nor should women be treated who have not fully recovered from childbirth.

(5) Severe heart disease, extreme fatigue or inebriation.

Chapter 2
Meridians and Acupoints in Brief

The theory of meridians and collaterals (energy channels and their branches) concentrates on the study of the physiological functions, pathological changes and the relations between the meridians and the internal organs of the body. Like the theory of vicera (theory of internal organs) and other theories of traditional Chinese medicine, the theory of meridians and collaterals is not an anatomical concept. Rather, it covers certain physiological and pathological ideas, as do most theories of traditional Chinese medicine.

The theory of meridians and collaterals is based on the accumulative experience of the ancient people and their doctors in combating disease over 2,000 years ago. In their long-term medical practice, the ancient doctors discovered the paths and various regular phenomena of meridians, including reaction points. Gradually they summarized, improved and developed their discoveries into a systematic theory. This theory not only provides the basis for self-massage along meridians and acupoints, but also guides all of traditional Chinese medical practice in its physiological, pathological, diagnostic and therapeutic aspects. Based on the studies of meridians and collaterals undertaken by doctors in earlier dynasties, Yu Jiayan, a celebrated doctor in the Ming Dynasty (1368-1644) pointed out in his book *Medical Principles*: "Ignorance of the 12 meridians will inevitably lead to errors in treatment."

The meridians and collaterals are the material bases for the transportation of *qi* and blood as well as various nutrients for the tissues and organs in the whole body. They are also the routes connecting and regulating the viscera, limbs, joints, the upper and lower as well as the interior and exterior parts of the body. The meridians and collaterals unite the viscera, limbs, all joints in the body, five sensory organs, nine orifices, skin, muscles, tendons and vessels into an integral whole. The meridians and collaterals can defend the body by resisting the invasion of exogenous pathogenic factors. However, when healthy energy (*zhengqi*) is deficient and pathogenic factors (*xieqi*) invade the body, meridians and collaterals become the routes for the transmission of pathogenic factors. When pathogenic factors attack the surface of the body, they can be transmitted through the meridians and collaterals from the exterior to the interior and from the shallow region into the deep region to invade the viscera. Since meridians and collaterals flow along certain regions and connect with certain viscera, they can manifest the disorders of the viscera along the reaction lines or points. So the manifestations of diseases, the meridians and collaterals and the connected viscera can be used as guides to differentiate diseases for the application of self-massage along meridians and acupoints.

Section 1 Meridians

Meridian is a collective term for both meridians and collaterals. Meridian means route and is the trunk of the meridian system; collateral means branch and is the branch of the meridian network, smaller than a meridian. The meridians and collaterals are distributed all through the body like an endless circle. This system connects with the viscera in the interior, associates with the limbs and joints in the exterior, uniting the body into an organic whole.

The system of meridians and collaterals is composed of 12 meridians, 12 branches, 12 tendons, 12 skin regions, eight extraordinary meridians, 15 major collaterals and numerous sub-collaterals. To be specific, the meridians include the 12 meridians, 12 branches of meridians and eight extraordinary meridians; the collaterals include 15 major collaterals, superficial collaterals and sub-collaterals. The tendons refer to the tendons directly related to the 12 meridians. The skin regions refer to the surface areas of the body over which the functions of the 12 meridians are manifested (Fig. 1).

1. The 12 Meridians

The 12 meridians are associated with the 12 viscera, and each of the meridians is connected with one of the viscera. The 12 meridians flow along the right and left sides of the body from the head, trunk and four limbs to the whole body. Since the 12 meridians form the trunk of the meridian system, they are called the 12 regular meridians. The 12 meridians are divided into two parts, i.e., *yin* meridians and *yang* meridians.

The *yin* meridians pertain to the *zang* organs (internal organs of the body, usually referring to the heart, liver, spleen, lungs and kidneys) and are connected with the *fu* organs (including the stomach, gall, intestines and bladder). Usually, the *yin* meridians flow along the medial of the four limbs as well as the chest and abdomen. The ones that flow along the medial side of the upper limbs (or inner side when the palms are facing forward as the hands hang at the sides of the body) are called the three *yin* meridians of the hand, while the ones that flow along the inner side of the lower limbs are called the three *yin* meridians of the foot.

Yang meridians pertain to the *fu* organs and are connected with the *zang* organs. Most of the *yang* meridians flow along the lateral side of the four limbs as well as the back, head and face. The ones that flow along the lateral side of the upper limbs (or thumb-side when the palms are facing forward as the hands hang at the sides of the body) are called three *yang* meridians of the hand, while the ones that flow along the lateral side of the lower limbs are called three *yang* meridians of the foot. The 12 meridians not only have their own flowing routes, but also are connected with each other.

The flowing directions of the 12 meridians, conceptions and governor vessels:

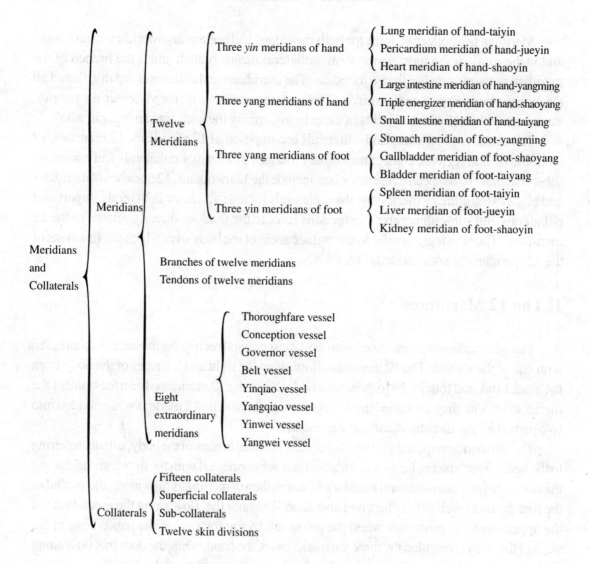

Fig. 1 The composition of meridians and collaterals.

(1) The meridians that start from the chest and flow to the hand are the lung meridian, heart meridian and pericardium meridian.

(2) The meridians that start from the hand and flow to the head are the small intestine meridian, large intestine meridian and triple energizer meridian.

(3) The meridians that start from the foot and flow to the abdomen and the chest are the spleen meridian, liver meridian and kidney meridian.

(4) The meridians that start from the head and flow to the foot are the stomach meridian, gallbladder meridian and bladder meridian.

(5) The conception and governor vessels all start from the perineum, flow along the anterior or the posterior midline from the lower part to the upper part (see Fig. 2).

2. The 12 Meridian Branches

The 12 meridian branches stem from the 12 meridians and function to reinforce the association between the meridians in relationship to the exterior and interior regions of the body.

3. The 12 Meridian Tendons

The 12 meridian tendons are attached to the 12 meridians. They are connected with the four limbs and all joints, and they govern the movement of the joints.

4. The Eight Extraordinary Vessels

The eight extraordinary meridians include the conception vessel, governor vessel, thoroughfare vessel, belt vessel, yinqiao vessel, yangqiao vessel, yinwei vessel and yangwei vessel, all of which are effective in commanding, associating and regulating the 12 meridians.

(1) The conception vessel: The conception vessel flows over the chest and abdomen and regulates all the *yin* meridians in the body. So it is called the sea of *yin* meridians.

(2) The governor vessel: The governor vessel flows along the back and regulates all the *yang* meridians. So it is called the sea of *yang* meridians.

(3) The thoroughfare vessel: The thoroughfare vessel flows parallel to the bladder meridian and is connected with all the meridians. So it is called the sea of the 12 meridians.

(4) The belt vessel: The belt vessel is distributed below the hypochondria and flows around the body like a belt. So it controls both the *yin* and *yang* meridians.

(5) The yinqiao vessel: The yinqiao vessel starts form the medial side of the heel and flows upward parallel to the kidney meridian, governing the movement of the lower limbs and

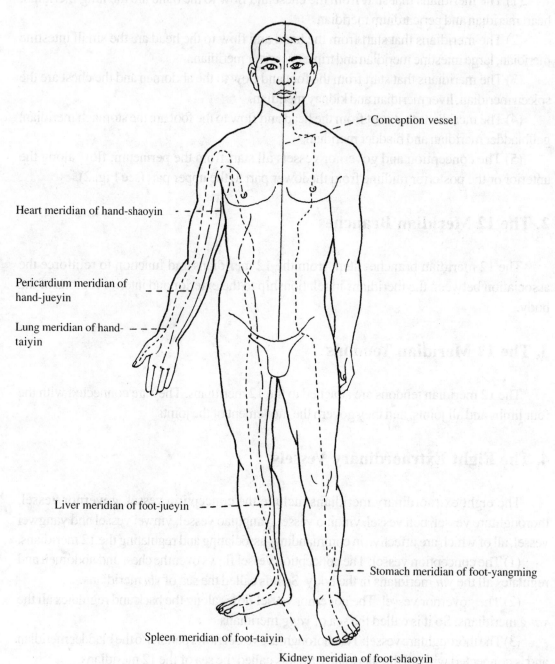

Conception vessel

Heart meridian of hand-shaoyin

Pericardium meridian of hand-jueyin

Lung meridian of hand-taiyin

Liver meridian of foot-jueyin

Stomach meridian of foot-yangming

Spleen meridian of foot-taiyin

Kidney meridian of foot-shaoyin

Fig. 2 Distribution of the fourteen meridians①

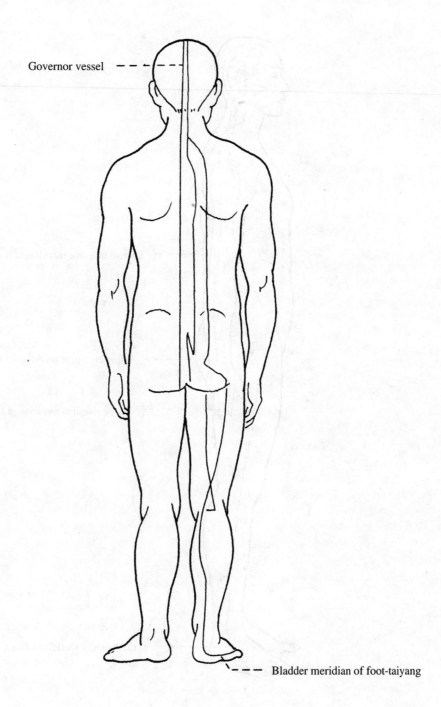

Governor vessel

Bladder meridian of foot-taiyang

Fig. 2 Distribution of the fourteen meridians②

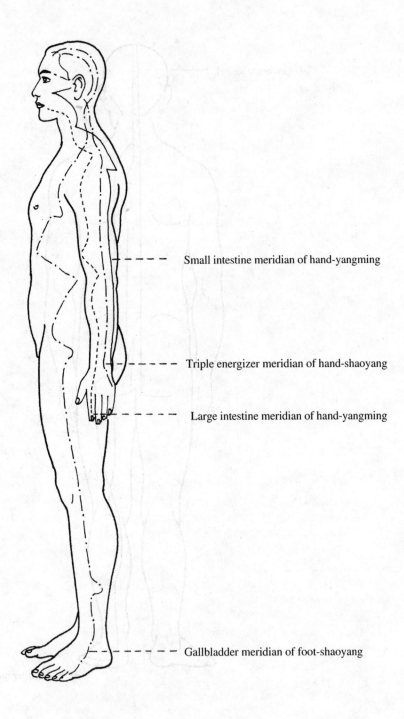

Small intestine meridian of hand-yangming

Triple energizer meridian of hand-shaoyang

Large intestine meridian of hand-yangming

Gallbladder meridian of foot-shaoyang

Fig. 2 Distribution of the fourteen meridians ③

sleep.

(6) The yangqiao vessel: The yangqiao vessel starts from the lateral side of the heel and flows upward with the bladder meridian, governing the movement of the lower limbs and sleep.

(7) The yinwei vessel: The yinwei vessel starts from the medial side of the shank and flows upward with the spleen meridian, controlling all the *yin* meridians.

(8) The yangwei vessel: The yangwei vessel starts form the heel, emerges from the external ankle, flows upward with the gallbladder meridian and controls all the *yang* meridians.

5. The 15 Collaterals

Each of the 12 meridians and the conception and govern vessels has a collateral. Together with the major collateral of the spleen, there are 15 collaterals in all. The function of the 15 collaterals is to reinforce the relation between the two meridians in exterior and interior relation over the surface of the body. The 15 collaterals also supplement the functions of the 12 meridians and the conception and governor vessels.

6. The Superficial Collaterals

The superficial collaterals flow in the surface areas and are usually visible.

7. Sub-collaterals

Sub-collaterals are the smallest collaterals.

8. The 12 Skin Regions

The 12 skin regions are the superficial areas of the body that reflect the functions of the 12 meridians, and they are also regions where the *qi* of the collaterals are distributed. So it is said in the chapter on skin regions in the "Basic Questions" of the *Yellow Emperor's Classic of Internal Medicine*: "The 12 meridians and vessels all refer to the divisions of the skin."

The 12 skin regions are defined by the range of the 12 meridians as they are distributed over the surfaces of the body. So it is said in the "Basic Questions": "The skin regions are determined by the routes of the meridians."

Since the skin regions form the exterior layer of the body, they constitute the body's system of defense.

Section 2   Acupoints

The meridians and collaterals are the paths that carry *qi* and blood. They are connected with the viscera in the interior and with the surface of the body on the exterior. On the surface of the body are acupoints, special areas where the visceral and meridian *qi* flow to the body's surface. So when illness occurs, massaging specific acupoints can cure various diseases by regulating *qi* and blood in the meridians.

Acupoints also are known as transporting points, tunnel points and holes. Acupoints are the areas where *qi* from the meridians and vessels infuse. The acupoints are located along the paths of the meridians. The application of massage to cure disease is usually done by regulating the functions of the meridians and viscera through the acupoints. So the acupoints are both manifesting points of disease and stimulating points for treating disease.

1. The Classification of Acupoints

(1) Meridian acupoints: These acupoints refer to the ones located on the 12 meridians and the conception and governor vessels. They form the major part of acupoints, of which altogether there are 361. The acupoints on the twelve meridians are usually symmetrical in pairs. However the acupoints on the governor and conception vessels are located along the anterior and posterior midlines and are singular.

(2) The acupoints on the eight extraordinary vessels: These acupoints have fixed locations but are not included in the fourteen meridians. They are acupoints discovered through clinical practice.

(3) Ashi acupoints: These are acupoints without fixed location or names. They are determined by tenderness or other pathological symptoms. These acupoints are the ones described as "taking pain as acupoint" in the *Yellow Emperor's Classic of Internal Medicine*.

2. The Functions of Acupoints

Acupoints are located along the routes of meridians and are closely related to meridians in their functions. Physiologically, acupoints transport, infuse, accumulate and emit visceral and meridian *qi*. Pathologically, points ache or become numb or otherwise sensitive along a particular meridian when certain meridian and visceral disorders occur. Self-massage along meridians and acupoints regulates the functions of the meridians and viscera to prevent and cure diseases through manipulations on the symptomatic points for reinforcing asthenia and reducing asthenia.

(1) Local effect: Massage on the acupoints is effective in treating diseases involving the local or peripheral tissues, organs and viscera around the acupoints.

(2) Distal effect: Massage along the fourteen meridians is effective in treating diseases of the tissues, organs and viscera far away from the route of the given meridian. It is even effective in treating diseases located far away from the route of the given meridian.

3. Methods for Locating Acupoints

The curative effect of self-massage along meridians and acupoints is closely tied to locating acupoints with accuracy. The following are some of the commonly used methods for locating acupoints.

(1) Finger-measurement for locating acupoints: Since the length and width of a person's fingers is usually proportional to the other parts of the body, self-finger-measurement can be used to locate acupoints.

① The width of the transverse crease of the thumb joint is taken as one *cun*.

② The width of the middle joints of the index finger and middle finger together is taken as 1.5 *cun*.

③ The width of the middle joints of the index finger, middle finger, ring finger and little finger together is taken as three *cun*.

(2) Features of the body for locating acupoints: Body features are taken as natural indicators for locating acupoints. For example, the point between the breasts is Tanzhong; the point between the brows is Yintang; the point in the medial depression of the brow is Zanzhu; the middle point connecting the tops of the two ears (on an imaginary line along the back of the head) is Baihui; the point on the end of the transverse crease of the elbow when bent is Quchi; and the point touched by the middle finger when the hand hangs down is Fengshi, etc.

(3) Bone-measurement for locating acupoints: A unit of length, determined by the length of various parts of the body, is taken as a standard measurement that can be used according to proportional calculations to locate acupoints on people of any age, height and constitution.

① The length from the lower border of the sternum to the middle of the navel is taken as eight *cun*.

② The length form the middle of the navel to the upper border of the pubic symphysis is taken as five *cun*.

③ The length from the anterior crease of the armpit to the transverse crease of the elbow is taken as nine *cun*.

④ The length from the elbow transverse crease to the wrist transverse crease is taken as 12 *cun*.

⑤ The length from the femoral trochanter to the lower border of the patella is taken as 19 *cun*.

⑥ The length from the lower border of the patella to the top of the external ankle is 16 *cun*.

Chapter 3
Methods

Self-massage along meridians and acupoints is a method of preventing and treating diseases. However, technical skill is a prerequisite, and skillful mastery of required techniques is very important in the practice of self-massage along the meridians and acupoints.

To direct the effect deep into the body, self-massage along meridians and acupoints should be persistent, powerful, even and gentle. This is according to experience gained over long years of practice.

"Persistent" means that pressure should be continued for a certain period of time; "powerful" means that the force of the touch should be appropriate to a person's overall health, the degree and nature of the illness, the affected area and the nature of a particular technique; "even" means that pressure should be rhythmical and moderate in speed and strength; "gentle" means that the pressure should be stable, soft and slow. The touch must be light but not floating, heavy but not sluggish and powerful but not rough. Any changes in pressure should be natural.

Section 1 Pressing

Pressing means to use the tips of the fingers, the palm heel or the palm itself to press the meridians, acupoints and other regions. Pressure is applied gradually and then maintained until sensations are felt such as aching, numbness, distension or pain. In performance of this technique, the part of the hand that presses the acupoints or meridians should be firm on the skin, vertical and without mobility. This technique can be applied to the whole body. It is characterized by its ability to soothe the meridians and activate the collaterals, regulating *qi* and stopping pain, eliminating obstruction and removing stagnation as well as regulating the functions of the viscera (see Fig. 1).

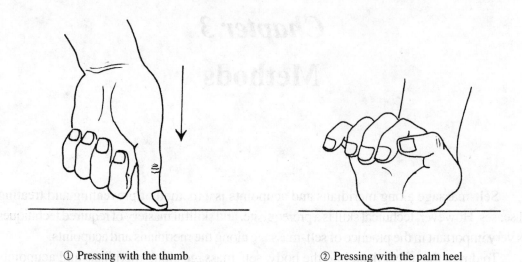

① Pressing with the thumb   ② Pressing with the palm heel

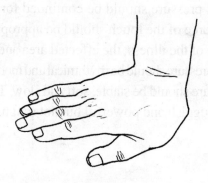

③ Pressing with the palm

Fig. 1 Pressing techniques ① , ② and ③

Section 2 Rubbing

Rubbing involves slow and coordinated rubbing using the fingers or palms on certain regions or acupoints in movements that can be linear or circular, clockwise or counterclockwise.

To assure comfort, rubbing should be neither heavy nor light but slow and gentle. The effect of rubbing can be transmitted deep into the skin. Commonly used on the chest, abdomen and hypochondria (the upper lateral region of the abdomen, marked by the lower ribs), rubbing is effective in improving circulation, subduing swelling, relieving pain, regulating *qi*, relaxing muscles and promoting digestion (see Fig. 2).

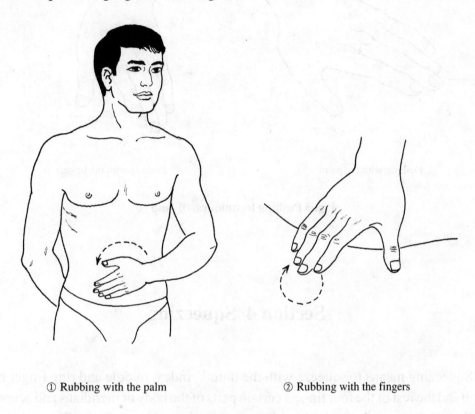

① Rubbing with the palm   ② Rubbing with the fingers

Fig. 2 Rubbing techniques ① and ②

Section 3 Pushing

Pushing — divided into thumb-pushing and palm-pushing techniques — means to use the thumbs or palms with gradually increasing pressure on certain areas and meridians. The strength used should be steady; the speed slow, even, rhythmical; and the direction, focused and linear. Pushing can be applied to the upper and lower limbs as well as the head, chest and abdomen. It is effective in dredging meridians and collaterals, softening hardness and dissipating nodules as well as in improving circulation and relieving pain. It is one of the most commonly used techniques for self-massage along the meridians and acupoints (see Fig. 3).

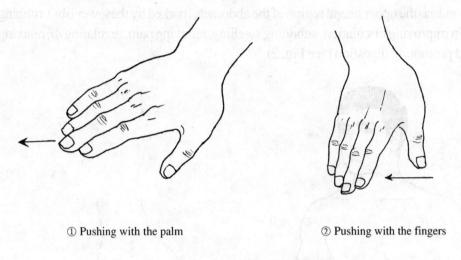

① Pushing with the palm   ② Pushing with the fingers

Fig. 3 Pushing techniques ① and ②

Section 4 Squeezing

Squeezing means to squeeze with the thumb, index, middle and ring finger or the thumb and the rest of the four fingers certain parts of the body or meridians and acupoints, usually in the area of the neck, shoulder, upper limbs and lower limbs. The technique is applied rhythmically with gradually increasing strength to provide strong stimulation. It is flexible but powerful. The pressure should be modified according to the situation. It is usually necessary to perform this technique until aching and distending sensations are felt. It is effective in expelling wind, dissipating cold, energizing the brain, stopping pain, soothing tendons and dredging collaterals (see Fig. 4)

Section 5 Kneading

Kneading means to use palm, or palm heel or fingers to press forcefully on the meridians, acupoints or regions from the front to the back, or from the left to the right, or from the

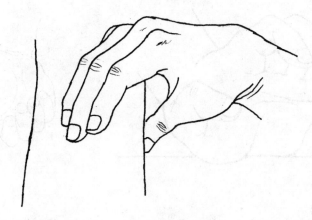

Fig. 4 Squeezing technique

shallow region to the deep region with soft, gentle and rotating pressure that moves the subcutaneous tissues. In performance, the fingers and palms should stick to the skin without moving around. The pressure should be rhythmical, gentle and soft to provide moderate stimulation. It can be applied to all the regions of the body, meridians and acupoints. It is effective in energizing the brain, refreshing the body, soothing the chest, regulating *qi*, promoting digestion, increasing circulation, subduing swelling and relieving pain (see Fig. 5).

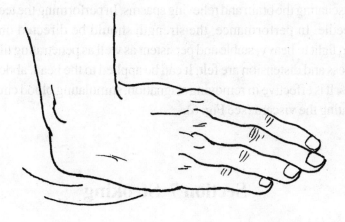

① Kneading with the whole palm

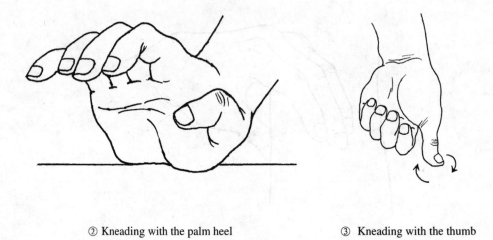

② Kneading with the palm heel   ③ Kneading with the thumb

Fig. 5 Kneading techniques ①, ② and ③

Section 6 Point-Pressing

Point-pressing means to press forcefully certain regions or acupoints with the thumb, or index finger or middle finger. The strength used to press is gradually increased, or the finger is pressed with a small rubbing motion.

Point-pressing evolved from the pressing technique and is usually combined with kneading. The area of point-pressing is smaller than that of pressing, but the stimulation is stronger. It can be used for resuscitating the brain and relieving spasms. In performing the technique, the finger is used as a needle. In performance, the strength should be directed on the vertical and moderated from light to heavy, stable and persistent as well as penetrating till the sensations of aching, numbness and distension are felt. It can be applied to the head, abdomen, back, upper and lower limbs. It is effective in removing stagnation, stimulating blood circulation, relieving pain and regulating the viscera (see Fig. 6).

Section 7 Stroking

Stroking means to use the palm and fingers to press on the skin over the meridians or

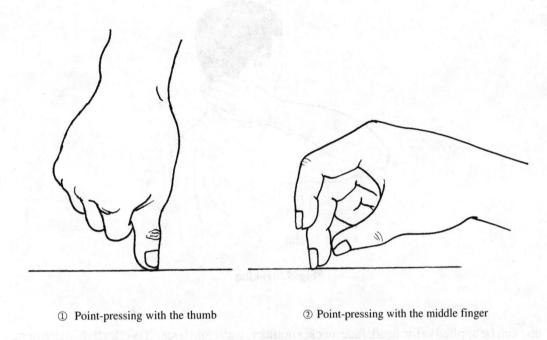

① Point-pressing with the thumb   ② Point-pressing with the middle finger

Fig. 6 Point-pressing techniques ① and ②

regions, gradually reinforcing the strength and doing continuous, linear and swift stroking from the upper to the lower or from the left to the right.

The pressure should be even and moderate to penetrate the skin and subcutaneous region till the sensation of warmth is felt. It can be applied to the chest, back, lower and upper limbs. It is effective in relaxing muscles, relieving fatigue, expelling wind and dissipating cold, warming and dredging meridians as well as promoting local blood circulation. It is one of the commonly used massaging techniques for self-massage along the meridians and acupoints (see Fig. 7).

Section 8   Pinching

Pinching means to pinch the skin over certain regions or meridians and acupoints, holding the skin up and rotating it. In performance, the technique should be coordinated, rhythmical and with gradually increasing pressure. The strength is concentrated on the tip of the fingers,

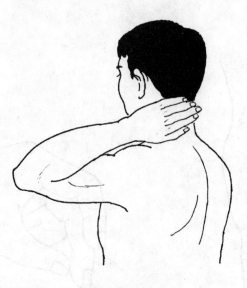

Fig. 7 Stroking

and can be applied to the head, face, neck, shoulder, waist and back. It is effective in dredging meridians, promoting *qi* flow and activating blood as well as relieving spasms and pain (see Fig. 8).

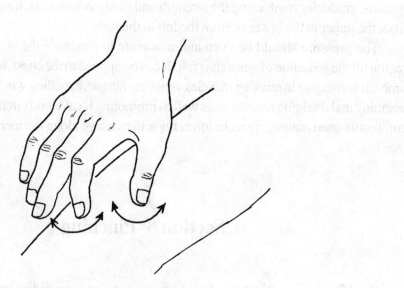

Fig. 8 Squeezing

Section 9 Pressing-Kneading

Pressing-kneading technique means to press and knead certain regions, meridians and acupoints with fingers of one hand or of both hands or with palms (see Fig. 9).

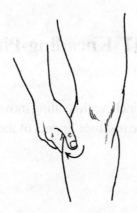

① Acupoint pressing and kneading

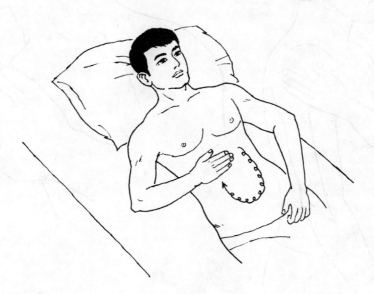

② Pressing and kneading abdomen

Fig. 9 Pressing-kneading techniques ① and ②

Section 10 Rubbing-Stroking

Rubbing-stroking means to rub and stroke certain regions, meridians and acupoints with palm or palms or fingers (see Fig. 10).

Section 11 Kneading-Pinching

Kneading-pinching means to pinch, with rotating movement, certain regions, meridians and acupoints with one thumb or the rest four fingers of the hand. (see Fig. 11).

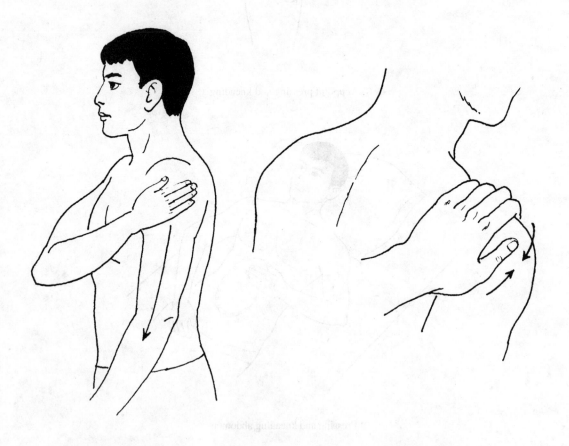

Fig. 10 Rubbing-stroking   **Fig. 11 Kneading-pinching**

Chapter 4

Healthcare

Section 1 Self-Massage Along Meridians and Acupoints for Strengthening the Body and Prolonging Life

Good health is essential to everything in life and work. So care must be taken to cultivate and preserve health. How to maintain psychological and physiological health? This requires one to be aware of and to follow basic healthcare principles.

As people become middle-aged or older, the functions of the viscera and the organs in the whole body begin to decline, as do the external functions of the body. Obvious manifestations are sluggish thinking, poor memory, slow reactions, poor hearing and vision as well as restricted movement. Self-massage (as well as massage done by doctors) along meridians and acupoints is effective in promoting blood circulation, regulating the digestive system, increasing muscular strength, lubricating joints, eliminating fatigue, invigorating the spirit, slowing senility and increasing the body's resistance to disease. Moreover, such massage — according to the traditional Chinese medicine theory of interior and exterior relations — improves visceral functions by balancing *qi* and blood, and *yin* and *yang* in the body to help strengthen body and mind in a way that leads toward achieving the goal of a long and healthy life.

Techniques for Self-Massage Along the Meridians and Acupoints

1. Rubbing the Hands

(1) Performance: Sitting or standing position. The palms touch each other and rub each other repeatedly, going from a slow speed to a rapid speed for about a half-minute. Then the right palm heel is used to rub the back of the left hand and the left palm heel is used to rub the back of the right hand for about one minute until a hot sensation is felt (see Fig. 1).

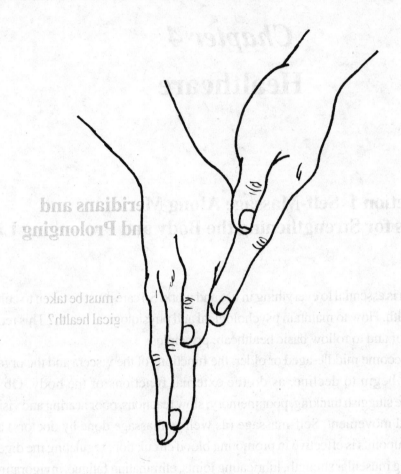

Fig. 1 Rubbing the hands

(2) Effect: The three *yang* meridians of the hand start from the hand and flow to the head, while the three *yin* meridians of the hand start from the chest and flow to the hand. So rubbing the palm and fingers can regulate *qi* and blood to make the fingers agile and dredge the meridians.

2. Rubbing the Face

(1) Performance: Sitting or standing position. First the hands are rubbed together for warmth before they are used to rub the face for about one minute in a washing motion from the forehead to the brows, eyes, nose, cheeks, the area in front of the ears and the corners of the mouth (Fig. 2).

(2) Effect: Traditional Chinese medicine holds that "the 12 meridians, 365 collaterals all

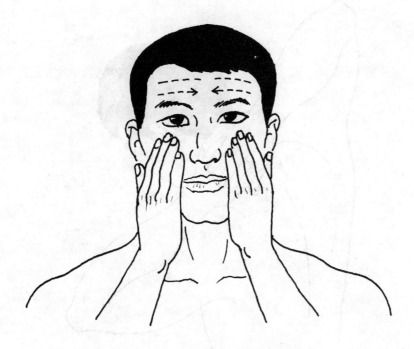

Fig. 2 Rubbing the face

transport *qi* and blood to the face and the upper orifices." So rubbing the face is beneficial to the functions of the viscera and the whole body as well as to the treatment and prevention of diseases. It is also effective in eliminating fatigue and refreshing the body.

3. Stroking the Back of the Neck

(1) Performance: Sitting or standing position. The fingers of both hands intertwine and embrace the neck. The head leans slightly back and the fingers touch the occipital region. Then the hands stroke the neck from the upper to the lower and from medium speed to rapid speed for about one minute until the area feels warm (see Fig. 3).

(2) Effect: The neck both supports the head and connects it with the body. The governor vessel flows through the middle of the neck. On the side of the neck flows the bladder meridian. Also, the neck is the important passage for the throat. So rubbing the neck can relax the joints, promote blood circulation in the head and face, strengthen metabolism, resuscitate the brain, brighten the eyes, relieve fatigue and invigorate the spirit as well as prevent and treat cervical vertebral diseases, vertigo and dizziness.

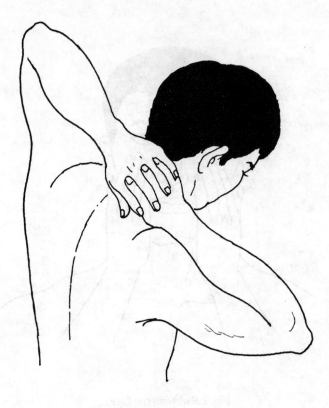

Fig. 3 Stroking the nape of the neck

4. Stroking Alongside the Nostrils

(1) Performance: Sitting or standing position. The thumbs bend slightly as the rest of the fingers fold into the hands to form soft fists. The dorsal sides of the thumbs are put 0.5 *cun* on the sides of the nose (Yingxiang LI20) and stroke along the nostrils from the lower to the upper with moderate strength for two minutes until the area feels warm (see Fig. 4).

(2) Effect: Stroking the nose can promote blood circulation in the nose, relieve cough and strengthen the resistance in the respiratory tract. It is especially effective in preventing and treating common cold and rhinitis.

5. Percussing the Head

(1) Performance: Sitting or standing position. The fingers of both hands slightly bend and stretch apart. The fingers tap the head from the hairline along the upper border of the forehead to the top of the head along the governor vessel, then to the hairline on the back of the head, the regions behind the ears and area of the temples for about two minutes (see Fig. 5).

(2) Press the index fingers or middle fingers repeatedly at intervals to help the nasal skin go up and down alternately. In fact, it is also effective for a number of nasal, eyes and mouth diseases.

6. Percussing the Occiput (the rear of the head or skull)

(1) Sit or stand, drawing in the chest, straightening your neck and lifting your head uprightly. Put your hands over your ears with the elbows raised and fingers pointed towards the back of the head. Then make the left and the middle fingers press the right ones, and press alongside the rear of the head.

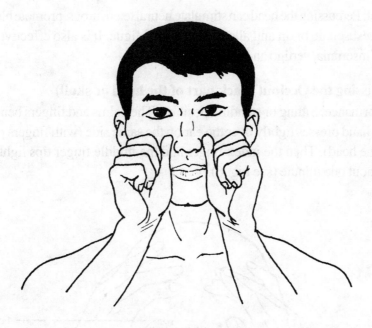

Fig. 4 Stroking alongside the nostrils

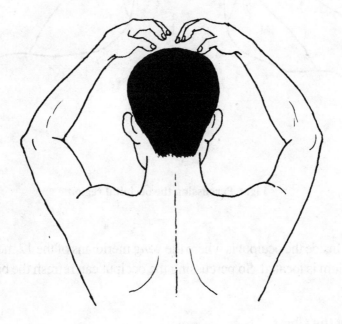

Fig. 5 Percussing the head

(2) Effect: Percussing the head can stimulate neural teleneurons, promote blood circulation in the brain, resuscitate brain and alleviate mental fatigue. It is also effective in alleviating symptoms of insomnia, vertigo and headache.

6. Percussing the Occiput (back part of the head or skull)

(1) Performance: Sitting or standing position. The palms and fingers bend slightly. The palm of each hand presses tightly over the ear on the same side (with fingers pointed toward the back of the head). Then the index finger and the middle finger tips lightly percuss the occiput for about one minute (see Fig. 6).

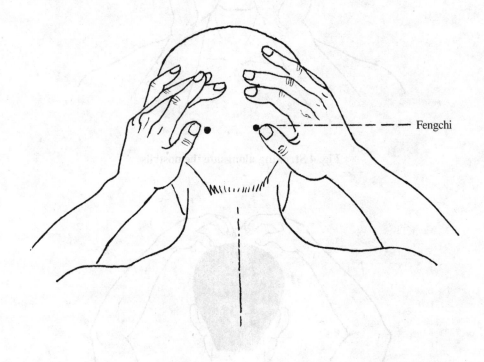

Fengchi

Fig. 6 Percussing the occipital region

(2) Effect: Inside the occiput is where the *yang* meridians of the 12 meridians converge and the cerebellum is located. So percussing the occiput can refresh the brain and improve memory.

7. Pushing the Chest

(1) Performance: Sitting or standing position. The palms and fingers of both hands push and rotate the chest alternatively. The right hand begins at the top part of the sternum

(breastbone) to its lower part and along the left side of the sternum to the shoulder and armpit for about one minute until the area feels warm and comfortable (see Fig. 7). Then the left hand repeats the sequence on its side.

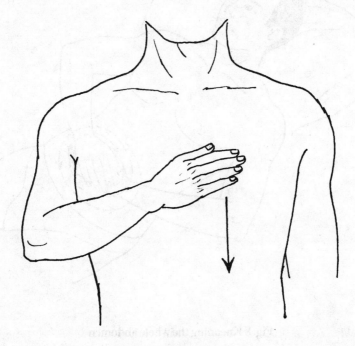

Fig. 7 Pushing the chest

(2) Effect: This technique can soothe the chest and regulate *qi* as well as soothe the liver and relieve depression. It is effective to some extent in relieving chest oppression and cough.

8. Kneading the Abdomen

(1) Performance: Supine position. The palm and fingers of the right hand are placed on the navel and the left palm and fingers cover the back of the right hand. The joined hands push and knead the abdomen around the navel from the right upward to the left downward. The kneading is done clockwise and gradually over the whole abdomen. Such a manipulation continues for about two minutes. The kneading should be moderate in strength and done until warmth is felt to be transmitted into the abdomen (see Fig. 8).

(2) Effect: The abdomen is the region where meridians converge. The conception and governor vessels are mainly distributed over the abdomen. That is why it is said "the abdomen is the palace of the viscera and the source of *yin*, *yang*, *qi* and blood. The viscera, limbs and skeleton of the body all depend on the cereal nutrients in the abdomen to provide nutrition. So

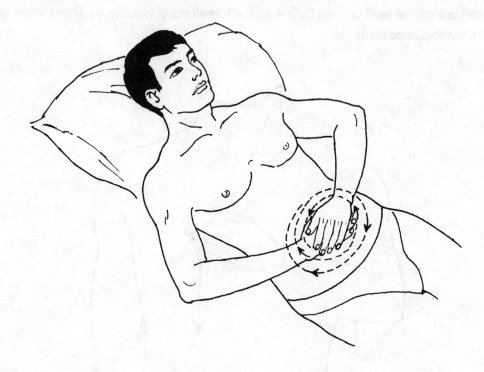

Fig. 8 Kneading the whole abdomen

kneading the meridians and acupoints on the abdomen is effective in regulating *yin* and *yang* of the whole body, adjusting the functions of the spleen and stomach as well as promoting the digestion, absorption and excretion of the body. Since the navel is connected with the viscera and can serve as a gate for the invasion of the pathogenic factors into the body, kneading and pushing the abdomen can boost the immunity of the body against diseases and prevent invasion of pathogenic factors into the body.

9. Stroking the Lumbosacral Region

(1) Performance: Sitting position. The palms and fingers of both hands are placed on the sides of the lumbosacral region and stroke forcefully from the upper to the lower for about one minute until the area feels warm (see Fig. 9).

(2) Effect: The waist is the region through which the belt vessels flow and in which the kidneys are located. The governor vessel flows through the middle of the waist. If the governor vessel flows smoothly, the kidney *qi* will be full of vitality. Frequent stroking of the lumbosacral region can increase vitality, primordial *qi* and kidney function as well as dredge the belt

vessel. It is also effective in preventing and treating seminal emission, impotence, irregular menstruation and lumbago.

10. Rotating the Waist

(1) Performance: Standing position. Stand with feet apart at shoulder width. The hands support the waist and the upper part of the body keeps immobile. The waist and the buttocks rotate together clockwise from the left to the right in a circle for about half a minute. Then the rotation is repeated in the opposite direction (see Fig. 10).

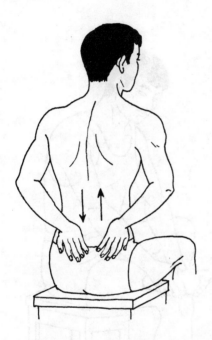

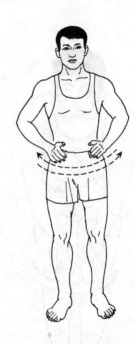

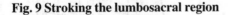

Fig. 9 Stroking the lumbosacral region   **Fig. 10 Rotating the waist**

(2) Effect: This technique can dredge the belt vessel, relax joints, revitalize the kidney, invigorate *yang,* strengthen the waist and spine as well as relax tendons and activate collaterals.

11. Rotating the Knees

(1) Performance: Standing position. Stand with feet together and the knees slightly bent. The palms and fingers of both hands are put on the knees and the knees begin to rotate clockwise and counterclockwise for half a minute respectively (see Fig. 11).

(2) Effect: This technique can dredge meridians, regulate *qi* and blood as well as relax joints. It is effective in preventing and treating gonitis (inflammation of the knee), paralysis,

numbness, weakness, fatigue and pain of the lower limbs.

12. Stroking the Yongquan Point (KI 1)

(1) Performance: Sitting position. In a seated position, the right foot is placed on the left thigh with the sole exposed and the entire right foot secured in place by the right hand. The hypothenar eminence (the fleshy edge of the palm under the little finger) of the left hand firmly strokes the Yongquan point (located in the middle of the sole in the area just below the ball of the foot) for about one minute (see Fig. 12). Then the same procedure is followed for the left foot.

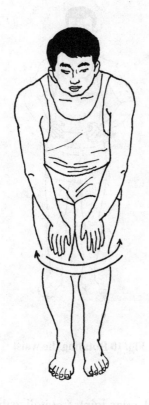
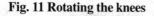
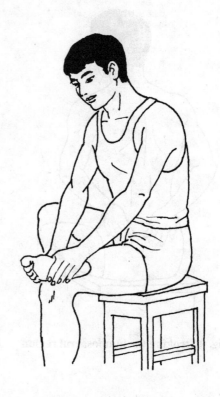

Fig. 11 Rotating the knees   **Fig. 12 Stroking the Yongquan point**

(2) Effect: The kidney meridian starts in the sole and ends in the upper part of the chest. Rubbing the Yongquan point can reduce asthenic fever [fever caused by a weakened condition, rather than an agitated (sthenic) condition] of the kidney as well as soothe the liver, regulate *qi* and brighten the eyes. It is not only effective in strengthening the feet, but also effective in

strengthening the legs and body to resist aging, improve sleep, prolong life and improve physical appearance.

Notes:

1. This 12-set application of self-massage along meridians and acupoints should be done once in the morning and once in the evening to both prevent and treat disease at an early stage. It is also generally beneficial in promoting health and longevity.

2. Self-massage along meridians and acupoints requires relaxation of the whole body, mental concentration and natural breathing. Each technique should be applied in a soft and steady way with strength. If the strength is too little, the technique will not work; if the strength is too much, the skin will be damaged.

The frequency and duration of massage should be decided according to an individual's condition as well as local skin reactions. The time can be adjusted and modified as necessary. Massage should last until one feels comfortable and relaxed.

3. Self-massage along meridians and acupoints requires persistence and determination.

Section 2 Self-Massage Along Meridians and Acupoints on the Face for Enhancing Appearance

The face is the region where emotions are manifested and where beauty can be revealed. So a face with firm and radiant skin is not only attractive, but also reflects a healthy body and a vital spirit.

When people are middle-aged, wrinkles begin to appear on the face, indicating aging and the decline of facial skin. This is caused by the reduction of subcutaneous fat and fluid, leading to malnutrition of the derma and a deficiency in the strength and elasticity of the skin. That is why the skin becomes flabby.

It has been proved that lack of proper maintenance and care of the face will lead to wrinkles even during youth. On the contrary, proper care of the face will prevent the appearance of wrinkles even in old age. So young women should be very careful about their face and take measures to prevent and delay the appearance of wrinkles. It is not right to think that it is useless to care for the face when you are old. If you persist in practicing self-massage along meridians and acupoints on the face, the blood circulation and metabolism in the face will be improved, making the face radiant, preventing aging and reducing wrinkles.

Techniques for Self-Massage Along Meridians and Acupoints

1. Rubbing the Face

(1) Performance: Sitting position. The head is straight, the whole body relaxed, eyes slightly closed and the mind concentrated on the region to be massaged. The two hands are rubbed together until warm, and the palms and fingers are used to rub the face (according to the description in Fig. 1) from the lower to the upper along the mouth corners, sides of the nostrils, cheeks, canthi (the angles formed by the meeting of the upper and lower eyelids at either side of the eye), forehead and nape. The rubbing is done continuously for two minutes (see Fig. 2). The hand movements should be harmonious, flexible, even and soft until the area feels warm, relaxed and comfortable.

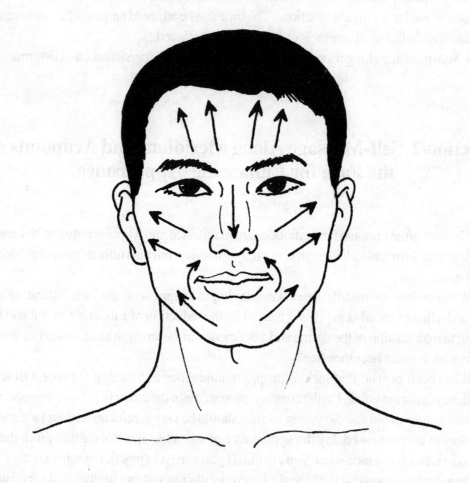

Fig. 1 Massaging directions

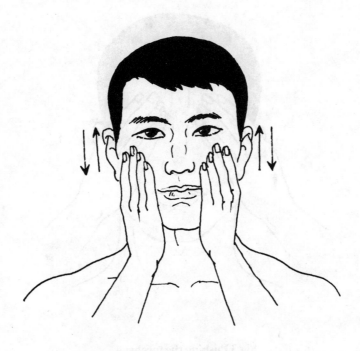

Fig. 2 Massaging the face

(2) Effect: Rubbing the face is effective in promoting blood circulation and metabolism of the face, making the face appear radiant, eliminating wrinkles and preventing aging.

2. Pushing and Kneading the Forehead

(1) Performance: Sitting position. The head is straight, the body relaxed, the eyes slightly closed and the mind concentrated on the region to be massaged.

① Pushing the forehead: With the index finger, middle finger and the ring finger of both hands held close together, the tips of the fingers are put on the forehead between the brows with the fingers pointing upward. The balls of the fingers push the forehead from the lower to the upper (to the hairline). The two hands then move to the Taiyang point (EX-HN 5) on each side respectively. This manipulation is continued for about one minute (see Fig. 3).

② Pressing the Yintang point (EX-HN 3): The pad near the tip of the middle finger of one hand presses on the Yintang point located between the brows and rotates for half a minute (see Fig. 4).

③ Kneading the forehead: The index and middle fingers of both hands are put between the brows to knead in circle from the brows to the Taiyang point on both sides for about one minute (see Fig. 5).

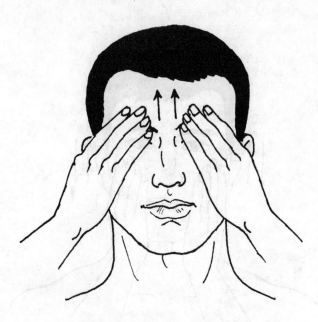

Fig.3 Pushing the forehead

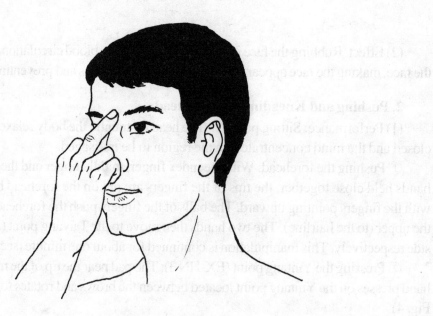

Fig. 4 Pressing the Yintang point

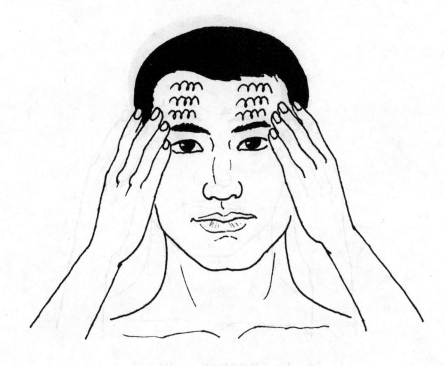

Fig. 5 Kneading the forehead

(2) Effect: This technique is good for refreshing the mind, brightening the eyes and preventing or reducing wrinkles on the forehead.

3. Rubbing the Eyes

(1) Performance: Sitting position. The head is straight, the body relaxed, the eyes slightly closed and the mind concentrated on the region to be massaged.

① Rubbing eyelids: The balls of the middle fingers of both hands are used to rub the upper eyelids from their inner sides to their outer sides and then to rub the lower eyelids from their outer sides to their inner sides for about one minute. The manipulation should be gentle and slow (see Fig. 6).

② Kneading the Taiyang point: The hypothenar (fleshy edge of the palm below the little finger) of both hands are put on the Taiyang point on both sides of the head (see Fig. 7) to knead clockwise for half a minute and then counterclockwise for half a minute.

③ Rotating eyeballs: The eyes stare straight and look upward, downward, to the left and to the right for half a minute.

(2) Effect: This technique is effective in brightening the eyes, reducing or eliminating wrinkles around the eyes.

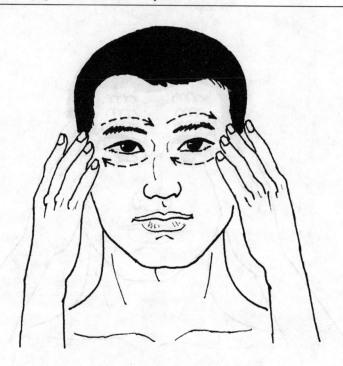

Fig. 6 Rubbing the eyelids

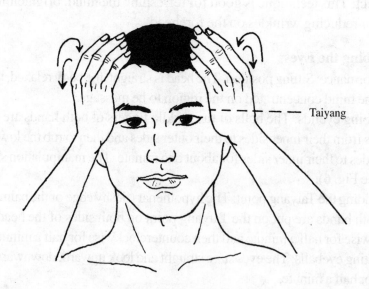

Taiyang

Fig. 7 Kneading the Taiyang point

4. Rubbing and Percussing the Cheeks

(1) Performance: Sitting position. The head is straight, the body relaxed, the eyes slightly closed and the mind concentrated on the region to be massaged.

① Rubbing the cheeks: The index, middle and ring fingers of both hands are used to rub from the mouth corners upward to the ears repeatedly for two minutes (see Fig. 8).

② Kneading around the mouth: The index and middle fingers of both hands are used to knead from the right corner of the mouth up around the upper lip to the left corner of the

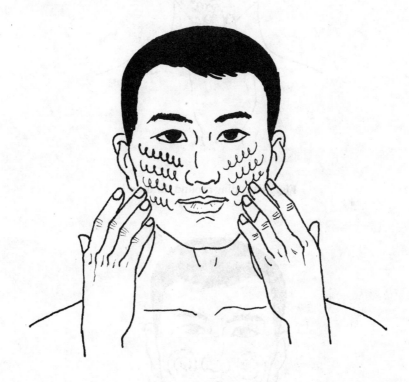

Fig. 8 Rubbing the cheeks

mouth, then from there down around the lower lip and back to the right corner of the mouth. This manipulation is repeated for about one minute (see Fig. 9).

③ Percussing the cheeks: The balls of the four fingers of both hands are used to percuss the cheeks gently and evenly for half a minute (see Fig. 10).

④ Pulling the lips: The mouth is opened as much as possible to separate the upper and lower jaw and make the lips tightly touch on the teeth. Then mouth is then closed. This manipulation is continued for about one minute.

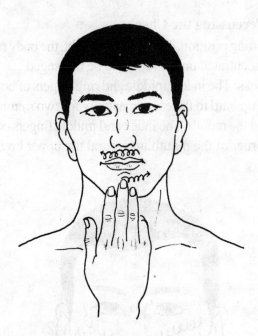

Fig. 9 Kneading around the mouth

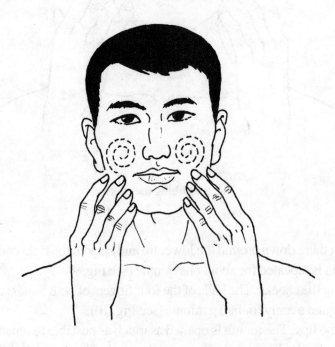

Fig. 10 Percussing the cheeks

(2) Purpose: This technique is effective in exercising the buccal (relating to the cheeks or the mouth cavity) muscles and preventing wrinkles and flabbiness around the corners of the mouth.

5. Pinching the Ears

(1) Performance: Sitting position. The index and middle fingers of both hands are used to pinch and pull the ears, especially the earlobes and tips of ears, for about one minute (see Fig. 11).

(2) Purpose: This technique is effective in warming and dredging meridians, regulating *qi* and blood as well as enhancing appearance.

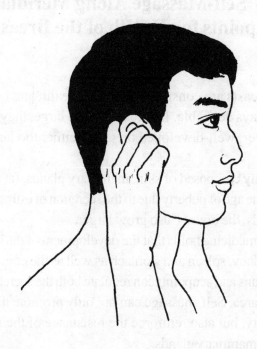

Fig. 11 Pinching the ears

Notes:

1. This set of appearance-enhancing exercises should be done with mental concentration, natural respiration and relaxation from beginning to end. The techniques should be accurate, flexible, gentle and slow. At first, the set can be performed in front of a mirror. Rubbing the eyes should be done with special care.

2. The order, frequency and time of performance can be decided according to individual

needs. Usually the set should be performed once in the morning and once in the evening.

3. The success of this set requires sufficient sleep, a regular life style, optimistic mood and appropriate physical exercise.

4. Also required: Rational diet, including foods with sufficient protein (such as soybean products), peanuts, milk, pork and fresh vegetables.

5. Be persistent and patient. Don't look for quick results.

Section 3 Self-Massage Along Meridians and Acupoints for Health of the Breasts

Full and shapely breasts are considered signs of health and beauty in women. But large breasts are not always desirable. If breasts are too large, they will detract from the body symmetry. However, well-developed breasts, neither too large nor too flat, often signify beauty.

The breasts are mainly composed of skin, mammary glands, fat and tissue. They grow larger when one reaches the age of puberty due to the secretion of estrogen. During pregnancy and breast-feeding periods, the breasts also grow larger.

Traditional Chinese medicine holds that the development of the breasts is related to the meridians of the liver, kidney, spleen and stomach as well as the conception vessel. So self-massage along the meridians and acupoints can regulate both the secretion of estrogen as well as directly stimulate the area. Self-massage can not only promote the development of the breasts to cultivate beauty, but also reinforce the resistance of the breasts to disease and promote the health of the mammary glands.

Techniques for Self-Massage Along the Meridians and Acupoints

1. Rubbing the Dazhui Point (GV 14)

Performance: Sitting position with the head slightly bent backward. The four fingers of the right hand close and put below the seventh cervical vertebral process where Dazhui is located. The palm and fingers are used to repeatedly rub Dazhui for one minute. The two hands are used to rub in alternation until the skin becomes reddish and feels warm (see Fig. 1).

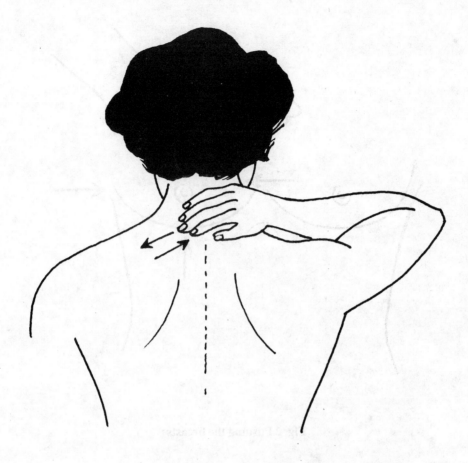

Fig. 1 Rubbing the Dazhui point

2. Pushing the Breasts

Performance: Sitting position. The right hand is used to push the left breast up toward the nipple, down toward the nipple, in toward the nipple and out toward the nipple for one minute. The manipulation should be gentle, slow and light (see Fig. 2). Then the left hand is used to push the right breast in the same way.

3. Stroking the Breasts

Performance: Sitting position. The thumb and the rest of the four fingers of the right hand are placed on the center of the left breast to stroke clockwise or counterclockwise around the nipple for half a minute (see Fig. 3). Then the left hand is used to stroke around the nipple of the right breast in the same way.

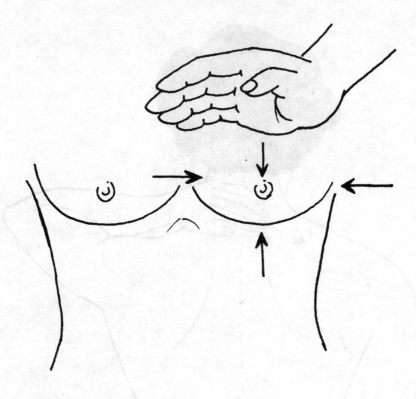

Fig. 2 Pushing the breasts

4. Pushing and Shaking the Breasts

Performance: Sitting position. The palms and fingers of both hands are used, with the hypothenar prominence (the fleshy edge of the palm underneath the little finger) of both hands holding the lower outsides of the breasts to shake and push the breasts up and down. This requires quick shaking with steady pressure. This manipulation is continued for one minute. It should be gentle and slow. The palms should not be higher than the nipple (see Fig. 4).

5. Adducting the Breasts

Performance: Standing position with feet shoulder-width apart. The palms touch each other and are put in front of the chest (see Fig. 5). Efforts are made to adduct (tense inward) and then relax the mammary muscles. This tensing and relaxing is repeated for one minute.

Then both hands are raised to the level of the chest (see Fig. 6). Concentrated efforts are made to adduct and then relax the mammary muscles. This tensing and relaxing is done for one minute.

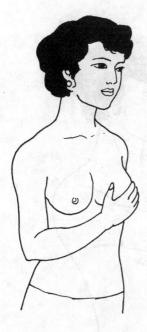

Fig. 3 Stroking the breasts

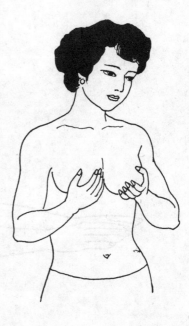

Fig. 4 Pushing and shaking the breasts

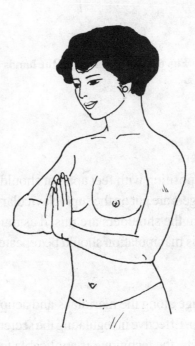

Fig. 5 Putting palms together

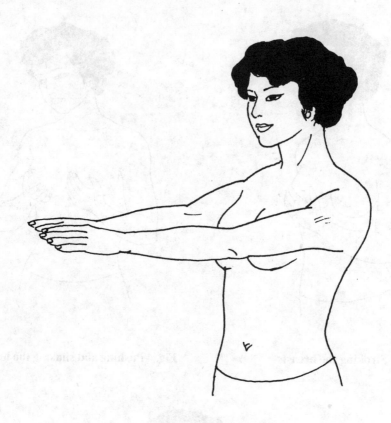

Fig. 6 Parallel raising of the hands

6. Raising the Shoulders

Performance: Standing position with feet apart at shoulder width. The elbow joints of both arms are bent and the fingers are put on the supraclavicular fossa (the shallow concavities just above the clavicle). Then the shoulders are raised as much as possible backward and upward and then relaxed. This manipulation should be repeated for one minute (see Fig. 7).

Notes:

1. This set of self-massage along the meridians and acupoints can be done once in the morning and once before sleep. Effective in regulating the secretion of estrogen and promoting the development of the breasts, the technique is applicable to breasts of any size or shape. Good results usually can be seen after two months of regular practice. There are no side

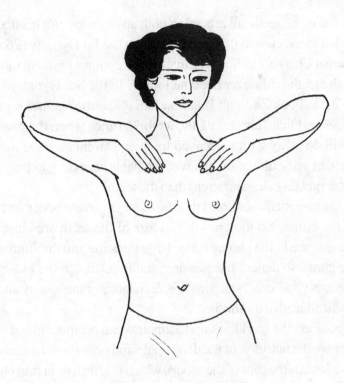

Fig. 7 Raising the shoulders

effects.

2. It is recommended that the massage be conducted in front of a mirror and without underwear. Skin Ointments or oils can be applied to the breasts for facilitating massage and a better curative effect.

3. Massage should be done with moderate strength and gentleness. Avoid roughness, pressure and squeezing.

4. Healthy diet and sufficient sleep are a must.

5. Push-ups, swimming, rowing or other such physical exercise is recommended.

Section 4 Self-Massage Along Meridians and Acupoints for Cleaning and Strengthening Teeth

Because the condition of the teeth play an important role in the digestion and absorption of food, healthy and clean teeth are crucial to both appearance and health. Ancient people paid much attention to the care of their teeth. Early in the Jin Dynasty (265-420), Ge Hong wrote in the "Internal Chapter" in *Bo Pu Zi* that "if one chomps the teeth three hundred times in the morning, the teeth will never become loose." In the Sui Dynasty (581-618), Chao Yuanfang wrote in his book *Zhubing Yuanhou Lun* (*General Treatise on the Etiology and Symptoms of Diseases*) that "chomping the teeth 36 times when the rooster crows in the early morning will do away with a decayed tooth and strengthen the teeth." Most of the masters in the field of self-cultivation believed that "it is necessary to frequently chomp the teeth" to prevent dental diseases and strengthen the teeth.

Traditional Chinese medicine holds that the kidneys govern bones and that the teeth are an extension of the bones. So the growth and loss of the teeth are closely related to the conditions of the essence in the kidneys. The large intestine and the stomach meridians are flowing over the gums, so dental diseases are usually related to the kidneys, stomach and intestines. Exogenous wind-cold, stomach fire, deficiency of the kidney and marrow as well as dental caries will all lead to toothache.

Self-massage along the meridians and acupoints can promote blood circulation, clean the teeth and improve the nutrition of the dental pulp and periodontal membrane (the portion of the gum that surrounds the root of the tooth), which is effective in preventing and treating dental diseases, atrophy of the gums and looseness of the teeth. Besides, it can increase the production of saliva in the mouth to promote digestion, remove toxic materials and boost immunity.

Manipulations for Self-Massage Along the Meridians and Acupoints

1. Pressing and Kneading Jiache (ST 6) and Xiaguan (ST 7)

Performance: Sitting position. The ball of the middle finger on both hands are used to rotate Jiache (ST 6) [located in the depression one finger above the mandibular arch (lower jaw)] and Xiaguan (ST 7) [located in the depression between the zygoma (cheek bone) and the mandibular notch]. Each acupoint is kneaded repeatedly for one minute. The manipulation should be gentle (see Fig. 1) (see Fig. 2 ① and ②).

2. Chomping Teeth

Performance: Sitting position. The body is relaxed, the respiration is natural and the mind is concentrated. Then the lips are slightly closed and the tongue touches the palate. The upper and lower teeth are chomped continuously, slowly and evenly. The front teeth are chomped for half a minute and then the back teeth are chomped for half a minute. Finally the teeth are clenched for one minute (see Fig. 3).

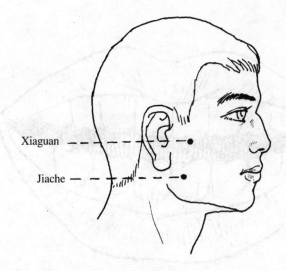

Fig. 1 Acupoints

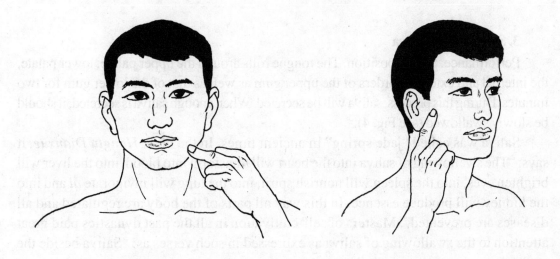

① Pressing and kneading Jiache   ② Pressing and kneading Xiaguan

Fig. 2 Pressing and kneading the acupoints ① and ②

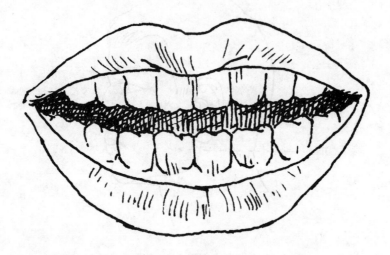

Fig. 3 Chomping the teeth

3. Swallowing Saliva

Performance: Sitting position. The tongue rolls around the upper palate, lower palate, the internal and external borders of the upper gum as well as that of the lower gum for two minutes. During this process, saliva will be secreted. When enough saliva is secreted, it should be slowly swallowed (see Fig. 4).

Saliva was called "jade spring" in ancient times. In the book *Honglu Dianxue*, it says: "The swallowing of saliva into the heart will transform into blood, into the liver will brighten eyes, into the spleen will nourish spirit, into the lung will invigorate *qi* and into the kidney will produce essence. In this way all parts of the body are regulated and all diseases are prevented." Masters of self-cultivation in all the past dynasties paid great attention to the swallowing of saliva as expressed in such verses as: "Saliva beside the teeth ensures longevity for me."

4. Kneading the Lips

Performance: Sitting or standing position. The thumb, index and middle fingers of one hand are used to knead around the lips (corresponding to the location of the gums) gently and slowly for two minutes (see Fig. 5). Then the other hand takes a turn.

2. To Rinse the Gum (Swallow Saliva)

Key points: Naturally close the mouth, use the tongue and both lips, agitate to form saliva until the mouth is full of water, then swallow it in dense, large gulps in sequence so that the region for swallowing goes to the chest cavity and the lower abdomen, with the swallowing sound heard (see Fig. 4).

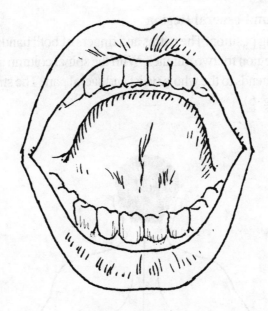

Fig. 4 Swallowing saliva

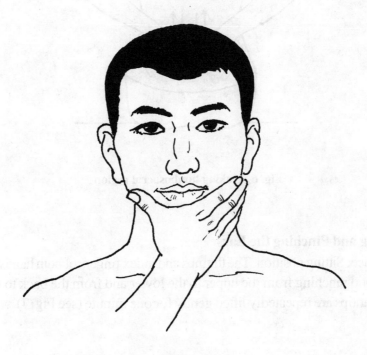

Fig. 5 Kneading the lips

3. To Knead and Pinching the Lips

Perfect action: Put the fingers together to form a pincer and with the pinching or kneading from the middle of the face and from the lips to the ears, knead and pinch gently in turn. Start from the center outward (see Fig. 5).

5. Stroking the Lumbosacral Region

Performance: Sitting position. The palms and fingers of both hands are used to forcefully stroke the lumbosacral region for two minutes. With the spinal column as the center, the region for stroking gradually extends to the whole waist and sacral part. The stroking is done until the area feels warm (see Fig. 6).

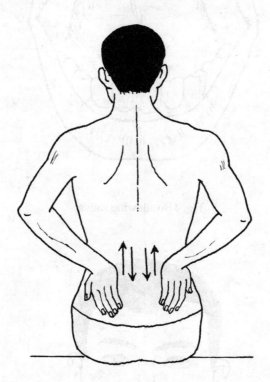

Fig. 6 Stroking lumbosacral region

6. Pushing and Pinching the Ears

Performance: Sitting position. The thumbs and index fingers of both hands are put on the ears, pushing and pinching from the upper to the lower and from the back to the front. The earlobes and ear tips are repeatedly lifted gently for one minute (see Fig. 7).

Notes:

1. Self-massage along meridians and acupoints should be done on a regular basis, once in the morning and once in the evening, for the prevention and treatment of dental diseases.

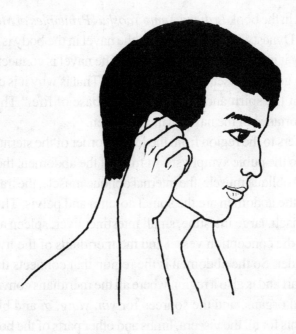

Fig. 7 Pushing and pinching the ears

2. Swelling and pain of gums accompanied by a discharge of pus should be treated by a medical professional.

3. Attention should be paid to dental hygiene; the teeth should be brushed after meals and before sleep.

4. Avoid too many sweets and eating before going to sleep.

Section 5 Self-Massage Along Meridians and Acupoints for Health of the Abdomen

Records show that self-massage along the meridians and acupoints of the abdomen to promote health has been popular since ancient times in China. In the Tang Dynasty (618-907), Sun Simiao's principle for self-cultivation was: "Walking one hundred steps after each meal and frequently rubbing the abdomen." In the Song Dynasty (960-1279), Lu You, a famous poet, often practiced an "abdomen-kneading exercise." Ge Hong, a master of self-cultivation in the Jin Dynasty, emphasized that "abdominal pain can be relieved by rubbing the abdomen." It was said in the book *Lizheng Anmo Yaoshu* (*Principles of Massage Techniques*) published in the Qing Dynasty (1644-1911) that "the navel in the body is like the Big Dipper in the sky. That is why it is called the celestial pivot. The navel is connected with the viscera and is the route for the genuine essence to pass through. That is why it is called spiritual gate. So it is the opening of the spirit and *qi* as well as the base of life." This description well demonstrates the importance of the navel in the abdomen.

The abdomen refers to the region from the lower border of the sternum (the lower tip of the xiphoid process) to the pubic symphysis. In front of the abdomen, the abdominal wall is formed by the external oblique muscle, the internal oblique muscle, the transverse muscle and fascia. In the back of the abdomen are the spinal column and pelvis. The viscera inside the abdomen are the stomach, large intestine, small intestine, liver, spleen and pancreas. In the abdominal wall flow the conception vessel and the meridians of the liver, spleen, kidney, stomach and gallbladder. So the abdomen is the region that connects the upper part of the body with the lower part and is also a region where all the meridians converge. Serving as the palace for all the vital organs, and the sources for *yin*, *yang*, *qi* and blood, the abdomen provides cereal nutrients for all the viscera, limbs and other parts of the body. So it is said that "the abdomen is responsible for the occurrence of various diseases, and the treatment of all diseases must focus on the treatment of the abdomen."

Self-massage along the meridians and acupoints of the abdomen for health can not only cure disorders of the viscera in the abdomen, but also regulate and invigorate all the tissues and organs in the body. It has been proved clinically that massaging the abdomen is effective in treating coronary heart disease, hypertension, diabetes, gastrointestinal dysfunction, irregular menstruation and menopause. It is also effective in preventing the invasion of pathogenic wind, cold, summer-heat, dampness, dryness and fire.

Techniques for Self-Massage Along the Meridians and Acupoints

1. Kneading Zhongwan (CV 12)

Performance: Supine or sitting position. The palm of one hand is put on Zhongwan (located four *cun* above the navel) to knead clockwise for one minute. This is done gently and slowly until the area feels warm (see Fig. 1). Then the other hand takes its turn.

2. Kneading Shenque (CV 8)

Performance: Supine or sitting position. The hands are placed on top of each other and put on Shenque to knead clockwise for two minutes. The manipulation should be light and gentle (see Fig. 2).

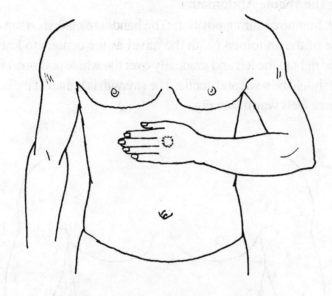

Fig. 1 Kneading Zhongwan

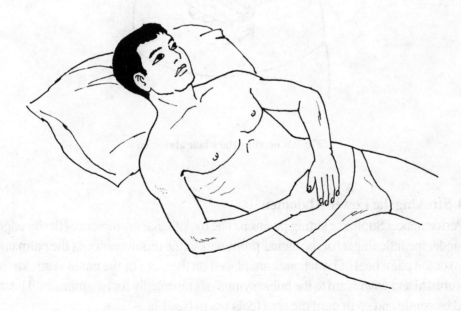

Fig. 2 Kneading Shenque

3. Kneading the Whole Abdomen

Performance: Supine or sitting position. The hands are placed on top of each other and put on the middle of the abdomen (with the navel as the center) to knead the abdomen clockwise from the right to the left and gradually over the whole abdomen for three minutes. The manipulation should be swift and gentle. The strength is lighter at the beginning and then heavier until the area feels warm (see Fig. 3).

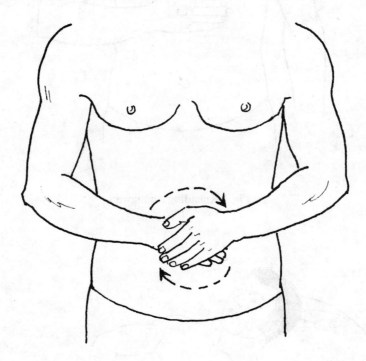

Fig. 3 Kneading the whole abdomen

4. Stroking the Lower Abdomen

Performance: Supine or sitting position. The hypothenar prominence (fleshy edge of the palm under the little finger) or the thenar prominence (the protuberance of the palm under the thumb) or the palm heel of both hands are placed on the sides of the navel to stroke from the groin forward and downward to the pubic symphysis repeatedly for two minutes. The stroking should be gentle and swift until the area feels warm (see Fig. 4).

5. Pushing the Conception Vessel

Performance: Supine or sitting position. The hands are placed on top of each other and put on the conception vessel to push and rub from the lower border of the xiphoid process to the upper border of the pubic symphysis with the thenar prominence (the protuberance of the palm under the thumb) for two minutes. The pushing should be heavy, slow and even (see Fig. 5).

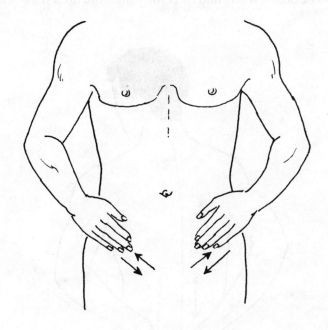

Fig. 4 Stroking the lower abdomen

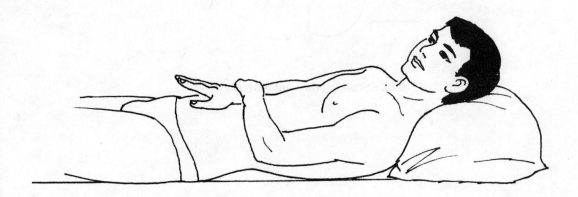

Fig. 5 Pushing the conception vessel

6. Stroking the Lumbosacral Region

Performance: Standing position. The two feet stand shoulder-width apart. The whole body is relaxed. The open hands are placed at the waist on both sides, with the fingers of each hand touching and pointed toward the spine. The palms and fingers stroke forcefully from higher on the back to the buttocks and from the buttocks up the back for one minute. This should be done swiftly and forcefully until the area feels warm (see Fig. 6).

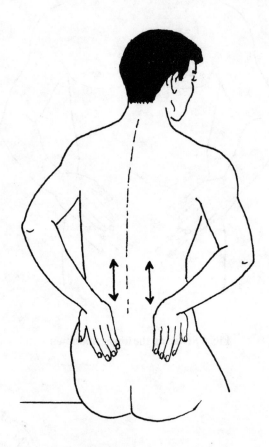

Fig. 6 Stroking the lumbosacral region

7. Rotating the Waist

Performance: Sitting position. The two feet are placed shoulder-width apart. The hands are placed on the knees, the whole body is relaxed and the respiration is natural. The upper part of the body rotates from the left to the right clockwise for one minute and then from the right to the left counterclockwise for another one minute. The range of rotation can be decided according to individual circumstance.

Notes:

1. Kneading of the abdomen can be done once in the morning and once in the evening every day according to the procedure mentioned above. The prone position is required, and the clothes should be unbuttoned. Kneading should be done with mental concentration and natural breathing.

2. Kneading should be gentle, slow, even and rhythmical. The amount of strength used should be determined according to individual circumstance. The kneading is continued until the area feels warm.

3. Do not knead the abdomen when feeling hungry or full or when the bladder is full. Kneading of the abdomen should be avoided if one suffers from internal bleeding due to gastric ulcers, duodenal bulbar ulcer or hemorrhoids. Rubbing the abdomen also should be avoided during menstruation.

Section 6　Self-Massage Along Meridians and Acupoints for Losing Weight

Being overweight is undesirable in people of any age. It not only affects appearance, but also affects the heart and overall health, making people vulnerable to heart disease, hypertension, diabetes, arthritis and angitis and other conditions that can be life threatening. That is why there is a worldwide concern about weight control.

Whether a person is overweight or not can be measured by his or her body weight. The medical criterion for standard body weight follows this formula: Male adult (kilogram)=height of the body (cm)$-100 \pm 10\%$; female adult (kilogram) =height of the body (cm)$-105 \pm 10\%$. If the body weight is 10% more than the normal standard, it is a sign of being overweight; if the body weight is 20% more than the normal standard, it is obese.

The causes of overweight are various, such as excessive intake of fat, disturbance of endocrine secretion, insufficient function of the liver and kidney, poor dietary habits and hereditary factors. Among these causes, excessive intake of food and lack of necessary physical exercise are dominant. If one lacks necessary physical exercise, the calories inside the body cannot be consumed and will transform into subcutaneous fat. The accumulation of surplus fat leads to an overweight condition.

Clinical observations show that a problem with weight in most (nine out of 10) overweight persons usually begins in the waist and abdomen. So methods of weight-reduction should start first at the waist and abdomen.

Self-massage along meridians and acupoints reduces weight mainly by stimulating local meridians and acupoints to soften and dissipate calories so as to reduce the accumulation of subcutaneous fat and promote the metabolism and consumption of fat. At the same time, it regulates the endocrine system, the viscera and the metabolism to reduce the accumulation of fat and strengthen the dynamic of the abdominal muscle.

Manipulations for Self-Massage Along Meridians and Acupoints

1. Pushing and Kneading Zhongwan (CV 12), Shangwan (CV 13), Jianli (CV 11), Qihai (CV 6) and Guanyuan (CV 4).

Performance: Supine position with relaxation of the whole body. The fingers of the right hand push and knead Shangwan (five *cun* above the navel), Zhongwan (four *cun* above the navel), Jianli (two *cun* above the navel), Qihai (1.5 *cun* below the navel) and Guanyuan (three *cun* below the navel) (see Fig. 1) for half a minute until aching and distending sensations are felt (see Fig. 2). Then the left hand takes a turn.

2. Rotating and Rubbing the Abdomen

Performance: Supine position and the relaxation of the whole body. The right palm is placed on the navel and the left palm is placed over the back of the right hand to rub and rotate clockwise for one minute. Then the rubbing starts from the internal part to the external part and gradually over the whole abdomen for one minute until the area feels warm (see Fig. 3).

3. Stroking the Lumbosacral Region

Performance: Sitting position, slightly bent forward at the waist. The five fingers of both hands are held together and placed on either side of the spinal column to stroke from the upper to the lower and from the lower to the upper. The rubbing starts from the middle to the outer sides of the back to cover gradually the whole lumbosacral region for two minutes until the area feels warm (see Fig. 4).

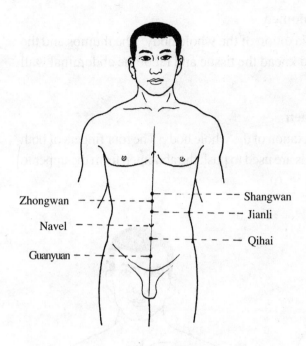

Zhongwan

Navel

Guanyuan

Shangwan

Jianli

Qihai

Fig. 1 Acupoints

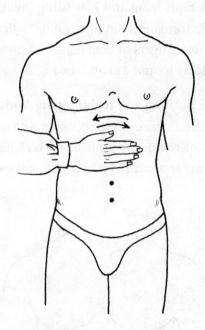

Fig. 2 Pushing and kneading the acupoints

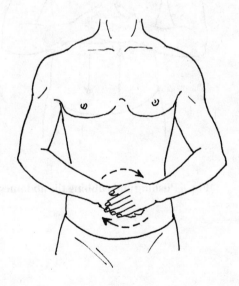

Fig. 3 Rotating and rubbing abdomen

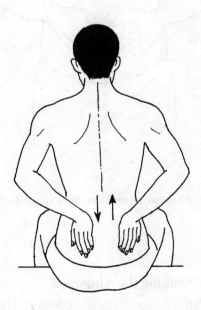

Fig. 4 Stroking the lumbosacral region

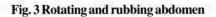

4. Squeezing and Kneading the Abdomen

Performance: Sitting position with relaxation of the whole body. The thumbs and the other four fingers of both hands lift up and knead the tissue and fat of the abdominal wall repeatedly for one minute (see Fig. 5).

5. Pushing and Rubbing the Abdomen

Performance: Sitting position with relaxation of the whole body. The four fingers of both hands intertwine and the palms of both hands are used to push the abdomen from the upper to the lower repeatedly for two minutes (see Fig. 6).

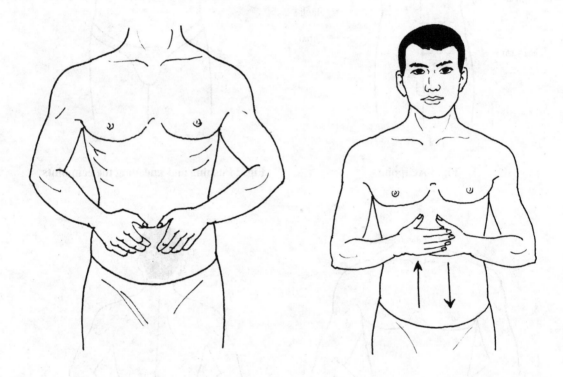

Fig. 5 Squeezing and kneading the abdomen   Fig. 6 Pushing and rubbing the abdomen

6. Shaking the Abdomen

Performance: Standing position. The two feet stand shoulder-width apart, and the whole body is relaxed. The palms of both hands are placed at the sides of the lower abdomen. The arms take the strength and quickly shake and vibrate through the wrists for one minute (see

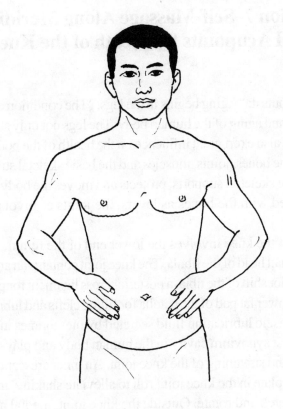

Fig. 7 Shaking the abdomen

Fig. 7).

The strength should be concentrated in the palms and fingers. The hands should not leave the skin and the shoulders should be kept still, avoiding pressure. This manipulation is effective in eliminating stasis and dissipating accumulation and relaxing muscles.

Notes:

1. The clothes worn should be of a thin material. The waist and the abdomen should be exposed so that techniques can be applied directly on the skin. Massage can be done in the morning and evening. Care should be taken to avoid becoming too cold.

2. The manipulation should be gentle and slow.

3. Frequent snacking between meals is a major contributor to obesity. Also, it is better to cut back on foods that are sweet, starchy or contain animal fat.

4. Physical exercise such as climbing stairs, climbing mountains and walking as well as squatting repetitions should be done regularly every day.

Section 7 Self-Massage Along Meridians and Acupoints for Heath of the Knees

As an old saying puts it: "Aging begins in the legs." The condition of the legs reflects the growth, development and aging of the human body. The legs not only support the movement of the lower limbs, but also exert great influence on the health of the body. The movement of the body depends on the bones, joints, muscles and the basic skeletal structure. Regulated by the nervous system, the skeleton supports, protects and moves the body. The activities of the body are accomplished with the bones as levers, the joints as pivots and the muscles as motors.

The movement of the knee involves the lower end of the femur, the upper end of the tibia, patella and the small head of the fibula. The knee joint contains an anterior cross ligament for preventing an anterior shift of the tibia, a posterior cross ligament for preventing a posterior shift of the tibia and a lower fat pad of the patella for filling clefts and lubricating the joint. The synovium (the clear, viscid lubricating fluid secreted by membranes in joint cavities) in the arthral cyst is the largest synovium cavity in the human body and plays an important role in enabling the bending and stretching of the knee joint. An inner crescent-shaped plate and an outer crescent-shaped plate in the knee joint roll to alleviate shaking, making it easy for the knee joint to bend, stretch and rotate. Outside the knee joint, medial and lateral accessory ligaments protect the bending and stretching of the knee joint to prevent adduction and rotation of the lower leg.

The center of movement for the lower limbs, the knee joint bears weight and moves frequently. With fewer blood vessels and fat tissue, the knee has an aversion to cold and dampness. It also is susceptible to being sprained. The quadriceps muscle of the thigh controls the stretching activity of the knee and is important for the stability of the knee joint. Care should be taken to train the quadriceps muscle of the thigh to prevent muscular atrophy and protect the functions of the knee joint. Frequent self-massaging of the meridians and acupoints around the knees and along the legs can not only regulate visceral functions and strengthen the knee joints, but also promote the circulation of *qi* and blood, nourish the tendons and bones as well as lubricate the joints. Massage helps prevent pathological changes in the knees and prolongs life.

Techniques for Self-Massage Along Meridians and Acupoints

1. Rubbing the Knee Joint
Performance: Sitting position, with the knees bent and lower limbs relaxed. The right

foot is placed on a stool. The fingers of both hands are slightly bent and the base of the palms rub the quadriceps in the thigh as well as the knee joint from the lower end of the thigh to the upper end of the thigh continuously for three minutes until the area feels warm (see Fig. 1). Then the left knee is rubbed the same way.

2. Pressing the Xiyan Point (ST 35 & EX-LE 5)

Performance: Sitting position. The thumbs of both hands or the thumb and index finger of one hand press and knead the Xiyan point located on the medial and lateral side of the lower border of the patella continuously for one minute (see Fig. 2). Then the other knee is pressed and kneaded using the same method.

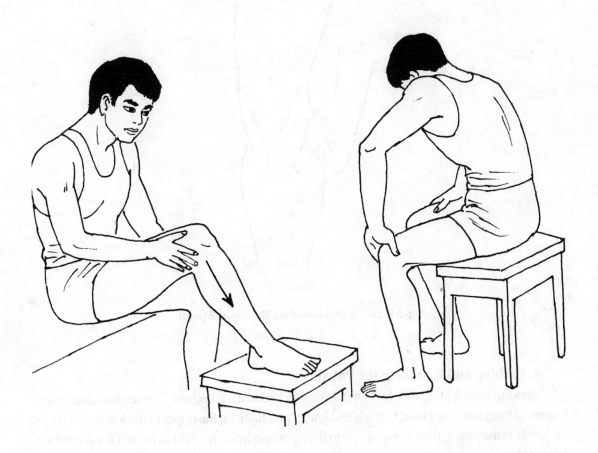

Fig. 1 Rubbing the knee joint   **Fig. 2 Pressing the Xiyan joint**

3. Pressing and Kneading the Zusanli Point (ST 36)

Performance: Sitting position. The thumb or middle finger of one hand is used to press and knead the Zusanli point located three *cun* below lateral Xiyan continuously for one minute until local distending sensation is felt (see Fig. 3). Then the other side is pressed and rubbed with the same method.

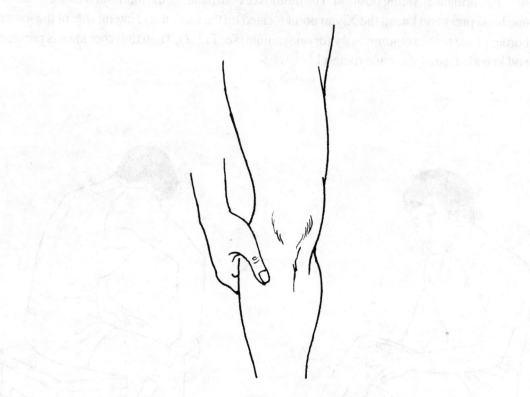

Fig. 3 Pressing and kneading the Zusanli point

4. Pushing and Kneading the Patella

Performance: Sitting on a bed with the lower limbs stretched out. The thumbs and index fingers of both hands are used to push and knead patella from the upper to the lower and from the lower to the upper, then from the left to the right and from the right to the left for about two minutes (see Fig. 4).

The palms of both hands firmly embrace the knee joint and knead for one minute (see Fig. 5). The massage should be gentle until a local warm sensation is felt. Then the other knee is embraced and kneaded the same way.

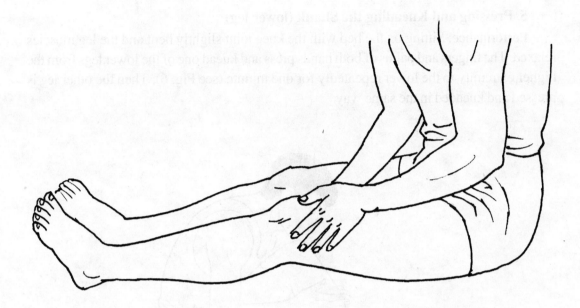

Fig. 4 Pushing and kneading the patella

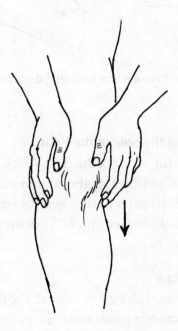

Fig. 5 Embracing and kneading the knee joint

5. Pressing and Kneading the Shank (lower leg)

Performance: Sitting on the bed with the knee joint slightly bent and the leg muscles relaxed. The fingers and palms of both hands press and knead one of the lower legs from the higher extremity to the lower repeatedly for one minute (see Fig. 6). Then the other leg is pressed and kneaded in the same way.

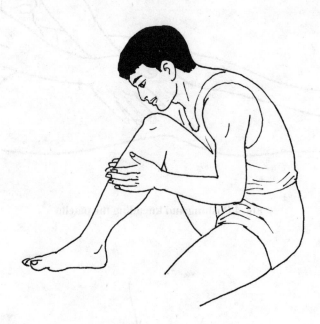

Fig. 6 Pressing and kneading the lower leg

6. Pushing and Stroking the Sole of the Foot

Performance: Sitting position. First, the right foot is placed on the left thigh. The right hand holds the right foot and the hypothenar prominence (fleshy edge of the palm under the little finger) of the left palm pushes and strokes the right sole repeatedly for one minute until the area feels warm (see Fig. 7). Then the left foot is pushed and stroked the same way.

7. Patting the Lower Legs

Performance: Sitting position with the legs relaxed. The fingers of both hands are slightly bent into empty fists. The hypothenar prominence and the lateral side of the small finger of both hands pat the lower limbs from the thigh to the ankle and from light to heavy for about two minutes (see Fig. 8). Then the other leg is patted using the same method.

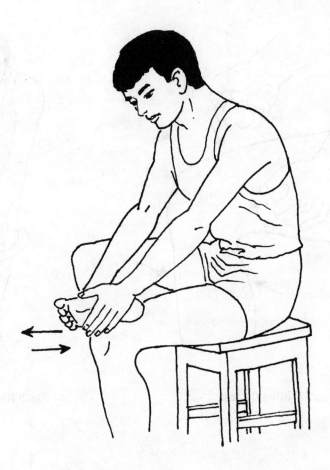

Fig. 7 Pushing and stroking the sole of the foot

8. Rotating the Knee Joint

Performance: Standing position. With feet together, the body leans slightly forward with the knees slightly bent. The palms of the hands are put on the knees. The knees first are rotated clockwise for half a minute, from left to right and back; then they are rotated counterclockwise for half a minute from right to left and back (see Fig. 9). The rotation range can be decided according to individual ability.

9. Kicking Movement

Performance: Standing with both hands on the waist or with one hand holding something for balance. The legs alternate swinging forward and backward for two minutes. The range is up to each individual.

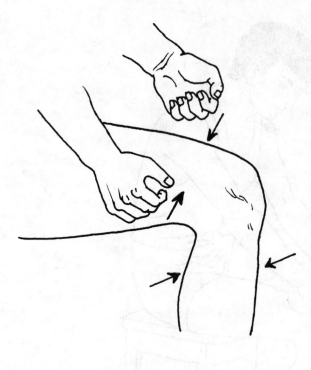

Fig. 8 Patting the legs

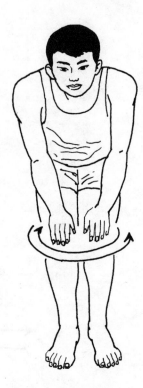

Fig. 9 Rotating the knees

Notes:

1. This self-massage along meridians and acupoints is done in the morning and evening every day. The massage should be gentle.

2. During the change of seasons, care should be taken to keep the knees warm.

3. Normal weight is best, neither too fat nor two thin.

4. Beneficial habits include taking a walk every day, slow running and stretching the knee joints.

Chapter 5
Therapeutics

Section 1 Common Cold

Introduction

The common cold is the most commonly encountered disease, an inflammation of the upper respiratory tract caused by a virus or bacterial infection. A cold can occur in any season, but especially in winter and spring or when people become weak and overworked. Colds can strike people of all ages and both sexes.

Traditional Chinese medicine holds that the common cold is caused by changes in the climate or a physical weakness, asthenia of pulmonary *qi* and invasions of pathogenic factors.

Symptoms of the Common Cold

The usual manifestations are a sudden onset with a dry and scratchy throat, stuffy nose, runny nose and sneezing — followed by sore throat, hoarseness, cough, headache, chills, low-grade fever and aching.

Application of Self-Massage Along Meridians and Acupoints

1. Stroking the Yingxiang Point (LI 20)

① Performance: Sitting or supine position. The thumbs of both hands are slightly bent while the rest of the fingers are folded into empty fists. The knuckles of the bent thumbs are placed against the Yingxiang located on the nasolabial groove (between the nose and the mouth) and stroke upward to the base of the nose and downward to the sides of the nostrils for two minutes (see Fig. 1).

② Effect: Self-massage along meridians and acupoints can improve blood circulation in the nasal region, increase tolerance to cold, strengthen the body's resistance, and treat and

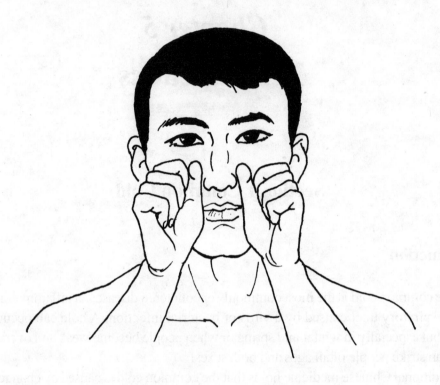

Fig. 1 Stroking Yingxiang

prevent common cold.

According to traditional Chinese medicine, the lung governs *qi*, controls respiration and the superficies and opens into the nose. The functions of the lung are closely related to the conditions of the lung. In the chapter of "Vessel Measurement" in *Ling Shu* (*Miraculous Pivot*), it is said: "The nose is sited in the middle of the face and is connected with blood circulation all over the body. The nostrils are related to the lung. *Qi* from the nose flows into the brain above and the lung below. So when the pulmonary *qi* is pure and when both *qi* and blood are circulating smoothly, no disease will be present. But when the pulmonary *qi* becomes predominant, it may lead to various diseases if it becomes stagnate."

2. Pressing and Kneading the Fengchi Point (GB 20)

① Performance: Sitting position. The tips of the thumbs of both hands are put on Fengchi on both sides of the occipital tuberosity. The rest of the fingers hold the occipital bone. Then both thumbs press and knead at the same time till local aching and distending sensation is felt. Then circular pressing and kneading is done from the inner to the outer side for about one minute (see Fig. 2).

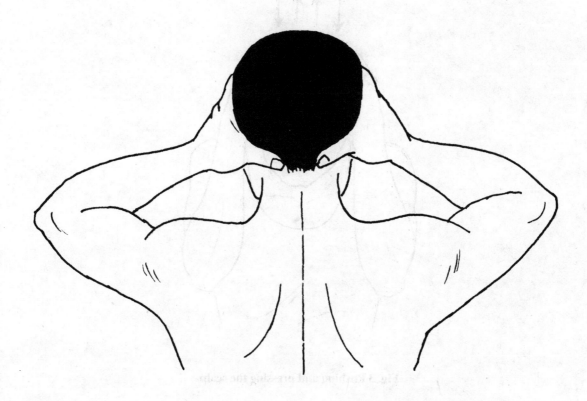

Fig. 2 Pressing and kneading Fengchi

② Effect: This method can help expel wind, refresh the brain and restore sleep. It can be applied to treat the common cold caused by exogenous wind-cold and exogenous wind-heat.

3. Pushing and Pressing the Scalp

① Performance: Sitting position. The fingers of both hands are slightly bent and forked. The finger pads are put on the hairline on either side of the head to push and press toward the crown until local aching and a distending sensation is felt. Then the fingers continue to push forward about two fingers-width at a time until the vertex or top of the head is reached. This manipulation is done repeatedly for about two minutes (see Fig. 3).

② Effect: It can stimulate the scalp and promote blood circulation in the head, helping to regulate the functions of the cerebral cortex.

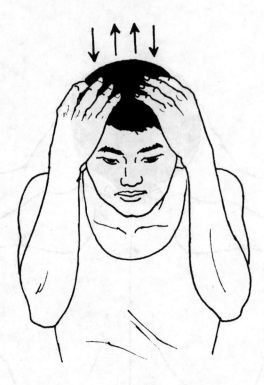

Fig. 3 Pushing and pressing the scalp

4. Squeezing and Lifting the Nape

① Performance: Sitting position. Both hands are rubbed warm and put at the back of the occipital bone with the fingers crossed. Then the base of the palms are used to grip the back sides of the nape, squeezing from outside to inside and then lifting up. This massage is continued for one minute until the area feels warm and comfortable (see Fig. 4).

② Effect: This method can help relieve spasms and pain as it dredges meridians and energizes the blood.

5. Pressing the Zusanli Point (ST 36)

① Performance: Sitting position with the knees bent. The thumbs of both hands press Zusanli located three *cun* below lateral Xiyan (ST 35) and one transverse finger lateral to the tibia. The pressing is done until the area aches and feels numb with a distending sensation (see Fig. 5).

② Effect: Zusanli is an acupoint used for healthcare. The pressing of this acupoint helps regulate the spleen and stomach, transform *qi* and blood as well as boost immunity.

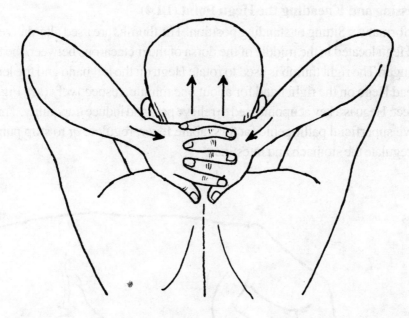

Fig. 4 Squeezing and lifting the nape

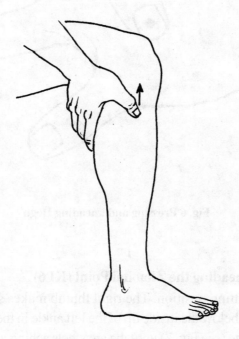

Fig. 5 Pressing Zusanli

6. Pressing and Kneading the Hegu Point (LI 4)

① Performance: Sitting or standing position. The thumbs are used alternatively to press and knead Hegu located in the middle of the dorsa of the metacarpus between the thumb and the index finger. The right thumb is used to rotate Hegu on the left hand and the left thumb is used to knead Hegu on the right hand for about one minute, respectively (see Fig. 6).

② Effect: Hegu is a key acupoint used to relieve pain and induce tranquility. This massage helps relieve superficial pathogenic factors, abate fever, regulate *qi* to stop pain, activate blood and regulate the stomach and intestines.

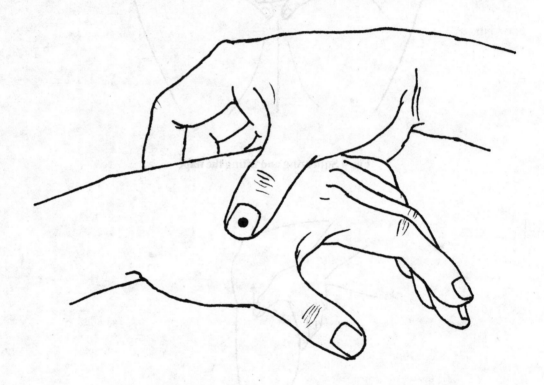

Fig. 6 Pressing and kneading Hegu

7. Pricking and Kneading the Zhaohai Point (KI 6)

① Performance: Sitting position. The right thumb makes small stabs at and kneads Zhaohai located one *cun* below the inside tip of the left ankle in the hollow below the border of the ankle for one minute (see Fig. 7) until the area feels aching and distending (see Fig. 8). Then the massage is applied to the right side.

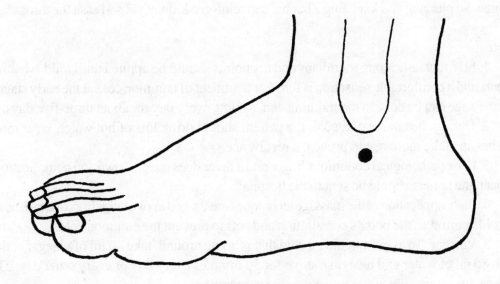

Fig. 7 Zhaohai

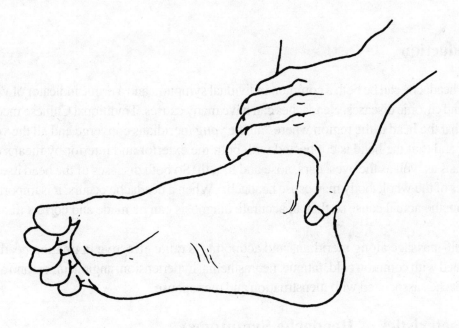

Fig. 8 Piercing and kneading Zhaohai

② Effect: Zhaohai is located on the kidney meridian that flows along the throat to the tongue. So piercing and kneading Zhaohai can reinforce kidney *yin* and ease the throat.

Notes:

1. Self-massage along meridians and acupoints should be applied until mild sweating occurs and a comfortable sensation is felt. For treatment of common cold at the early stages, the massage can be done in the morning and evening every day for about three-five days.

2. During the course of a cold, the patient should drink lots of hot water, wear more clothes and take more rest to prevent a recurrence.

3. If the pathological conditions linger and a fever does not go down and complications appear, the patient should be sent to the hospital.

4. Daily application of the massage techniques mentioned above helps improve resistance to cold, reinforces the body's constitution and acts to prevent the common cold.

5. Vinegar: To avoid catching a cold that is going around, take 40 ml of vinegar added with 80 ml of water and heat on a stove for 30 minutes every day or every other day. The vinegar fumes are effective in preventing the common cold.

Section 2 Headache

Introduction

A headache can be both a common individual symptom and a prime indicator of various acute and chronic diseases. Headaches can have many causes. Traditional Chinese medicine holds that the head is the region where "all the *yang* meridians converge and all the vessels reach" and that the head is connected with both the exterior and interior by means of the meridians as well as the eyes, ears, nose and mouth. So both diseases of the head itself and diseases of the whole body may cause headache. When a headache occurs, it is important to ascertain the actual cause so that an accurate diagnosis can be made and correct treatment applied.

Self-massage along meridians and acupoints is quite effective in treating headaches associated with common cold, fatigue, neurasthenia, hypertension, angioneurosis and as well as headaches associated with menstruation and menopause.

Characteristics of Headache Symptoms

The symptoms of a headache can vary according to the cause. The usual manifestation is a swollen and heavy discomfort in the head involving either a certain part of the head or the whole head. A headache can be accompanied by dull pain, piercing pain, drilling pain, throbbing pain or even swelling pain as in a "splitting" headache. The attack can be routine or continuous or periodic. Usually a headache is accompanied by feelings such as restlessness, fatigue, tinnitus, vertigo, nausea and insomnia, etc.

Self-Massage Along Meridians and Acupoints

1. Piercing and Pressing the Baihui Point (GV 20)

Performance: Sitting position with the whole body relaxed. The ball of the middle finger of one hand is used to press into the Baihui point located on the vertex for about one minute until a numb and distending sensation is felt there (see Fig. 1).

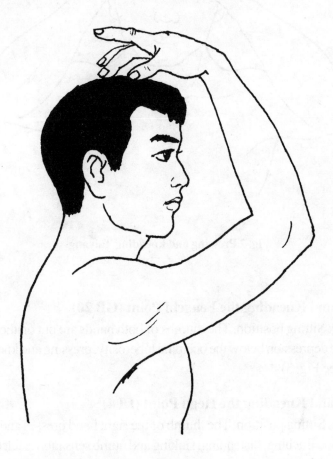

Fig. 1 Piercing and pressing the Baihui point

2. Pressing and Kneading the Taiyang Point (EX-HN 5)

Performance: Sitting position with a relaxed body. The hypothenar eminences (the fleshy edge of the palm under the little finger) of both hands are put on both sides of Taiyang located in the depression behind the middle point of the line between the end of the eyebrow and the outer canthus. Then knead clockwise for about half a minute and counterclockwise for another half a minute (see Fig. 2).

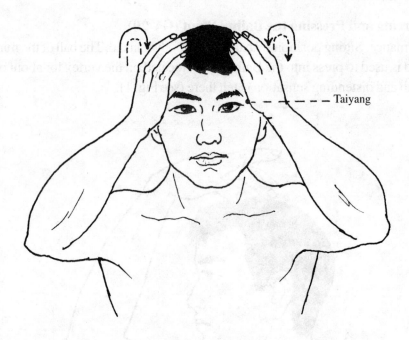

Taiyang

Fig. 2 Pressing and kneading Taiyang

3. Pressing and Kneading the Fengchi Point (GB 20)

Performance: Sitting position. The thumbs of both hands are put on the Fengchi on both sides located in the depression below the occipital tuberosity, pressing and kneading repeatedly for one minute (see Fig. 3).

4. Pressing and Kneading the Hegu Point (LI 4)

Performance: Sitting position. The thumb of the right hand presses and kneads Hegu on the left hand until local aching, distending, sinking and numb sensation is felt (see Fig. 4). Then the thumb of the left hand is used to press and knead Hegu on the right hand with the same method.

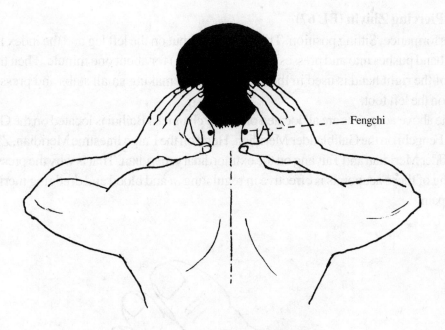

Fengchi

Fig. 3 Pressing and kneading Fengchi

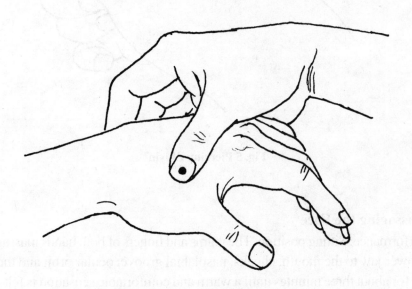

Fig. 4 Pressing and kneading Hegu

5. Piercing Zhiyin (BL 67)

Performance: Sitting position. The right foot is put on the left leg and the index finger of the left hand pushes into and presses Zhiyin (see Fig. 5) for about one minute. Then the index finger of the right hand is used in the same way with making small stabs and pressing into Zhiyin on the left foot.

The above acupoints are all located on major channels: Baihui is located on the Governor Vessel, Fengchi on the Gallbladder Meridian, Hegu on the Large Intestine Meridian, Zhiyin on the Bladder Meridian and Taiyang on the extraordinary meridian. That is why the pressing and kneading of these acupoints is effective in regulating *qi* and blood and dredging meridians to relieve pain.

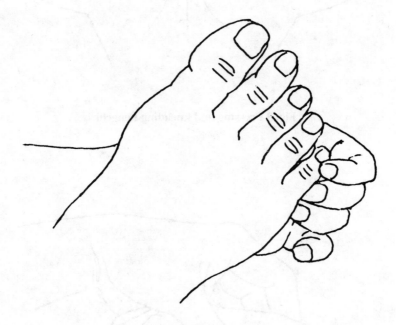

Fig. 5 Piercing Zhiyin

6. Massaging the Face

① Performance: Sitting position. The palms and fingers of both hands massage the face from the lower jaw to the mouth, cheeks, nasolabial groove, ocular orbit and the forehead repeatedly for about three minutes until a warm and comfortable sensation is felt in the area (see Fig. 6).

② Effect: This method can refresh the brain and brighten the eyes.

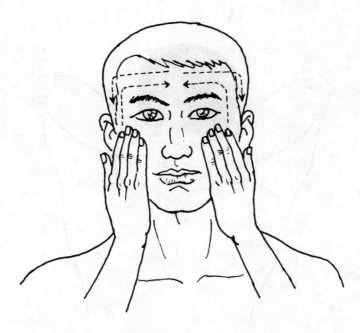

Fig. 6 Massaging the face

7. Squeezing and Lifting the Nape

① Performance: Sitting position. The hands are crossed to hold the nape and then the head is slightly bent back. Then the palm heels are used to squeeze and lift the nape repeatedly for one minute (see Fig. 7).

② Effect: This method can dredge meridians and activate blood as well as relieve spasms and pain.

8. Stroking the Nose

① Performance: Sitting position. The thumbs of both hands are slightly bent and the other fingers folded into empty fists. The knuckles of the bent thumbs are put at the sides of the nose to stroke upward to the skull and downward to the sides of the nostrils repeatedly for about one minute (see Fig. 8).

② Effect: This method may help dredge the nostrils and disperse wind and heat.

9. Percussing the Head

① Performance: Sitting position. The fingers of both hands are slightly bent and naturally stretched. The tips of the fingers of both hands simultaneously or alternatively percuss the scalp within the hairline for about two minutes (see Fig. 9).

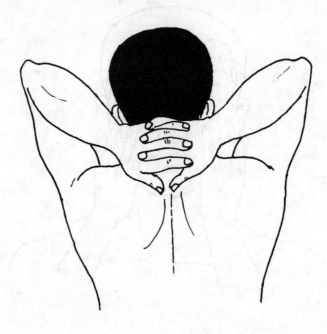

Fig. 7 Squeezing and lifting the nape

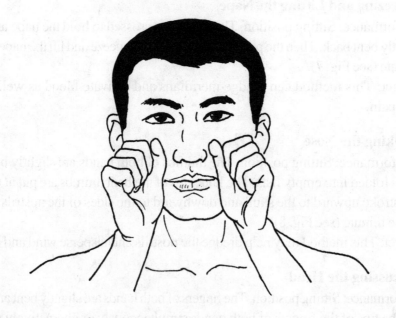

Fig. 8 Stroking the nose

The percussion is light at first and then gradually heavier until a comfortable sensation is felt and the headache is clearly alleviated.

② Effect: This method can activate the blood, eliminate stagnation and relieve pain.

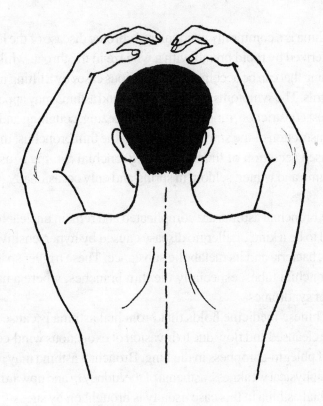

Fig. 9 Percussing the head

Notes:

1. Self-massage along meridians and acupoints for headache can be applied once a day. The frequency may be increased according to the location of the headache. The performance of the techniques depends on relaxation of the body, especially the head and the mind. Patients can be helped by keeping an optimistic outlook while avoiding overextending themselves.

2. If the headache is recurrent and cannot be relieved by techniques used in self-massage along meridians and acupoints, the patient should be sent to the hospital for further examination.

3. Daily life must be regular, and steps taken to avoid stress.

4. Also important: Proper physical exercise and the avoidance of mental agitation.

Section 3 Bronchial Asthma

Introduction

Bronchial asthma is a commonly encountered chronic disease of the lungs. Dyspnea (air hunger) is characterized by rapid breath with a wheeze in the throat, while asthma involves difficulty in breathing that can be accompanied in serious cases by a lifting in the shoulders and a flaring of the nostrils. The symptoms of both dyspnea and asthma may appear simultaneously. Symptoms like chest constriction, rapid breathing, wheezing, coughing and expectoration can be attributed to constriction of the smooth muscles in the thin bronchus, mucous congestion, edema and increased secretion of the bronchus. Bronchial asthma is usually seasonal — found often in autumn and winter, seldom in spring and only occasionally or much relieved in summer.

The causes of bronchial asthma are complicated and remain unclear to this day. But it is generally believed to be a kind of allergic disease caused by hypersensitivity to pollen, dust, paint, fish, shrimp, bacteria and its metabolic substance. These trigger spasms of the smooth muscles of the bronchial tubes, especially the thin branches, where a narrowing of ducts results in a series of syndromes.

Traditional Chinese medicine holds that bronchial asthma is caused by failure of the pulmonary *qi* to be cleansed and flow due to invasion of exogenous wind-cold into the lung or an accumulation of phlegm-dampness in the lung. Bronchial asthma may also be caused by a lingering disease or physical weakness, asthenia of the kidney *qi* and upward floating of various kinds of *qi*. Bronchial asthma in this case usually is brought on by stress.

Symptoms of Bronchial Asthma

The warning symptoms include nasal itching, runny nose, sneezing and general discomfort. These are followed by tightness in the chest, labored breathing, asthma, coughing and expectoration. An asthma attack may last a long or short time. The symptoms in serious cases are opening of the mouth, lifting of the shoulders, inability to lie flat, profuse sweating, cold limbs, pale lips and bulging veins in the neck. A patient usually feels weak and dispirited.

Manipulations for Self-Massage Along Meridians and Acupoints

1. Pressing the Danzhong Point (CV 17)

Performance: Sitting position. The tip of the middle finger of one hand is used to press

Danzhong located on the anterior midline, parallel to the fourth costal space, i.e., the middle point between the breasts. The pressing is continued for one minute until local aching and distending sensation is felt (see Fig. 1).

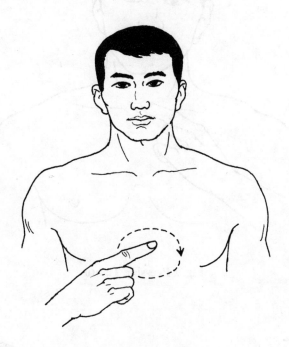

Fig. 1 Pressing Danzhong

2. Pressing the Tiantu Point (CV 22)

Performance: Sitting position. The tip of the middle finger of one hand is used to press Tiantu located on the suprasternal fossa (depression above the sternum) for about one minute until local aching and distending sensation is felt.

3. Pressing the Tianfu Point(LU 3)

Performance: Sitting position. One thumb is used to press Tianfu (see Fig. 3) located three *cun* below the axillary crease of the upper arm, i.e., the lateral side of the biceps along the humerus for one minute until local aching and distending sensation is felt (see Fig. 4). Then the other side is pressed with the same method.

Danzhong and Tiantu are located on the conception vessel while Tianfu is located on the lung meridian. This technique is effective in dredging meridians and tranquilizing the mind.

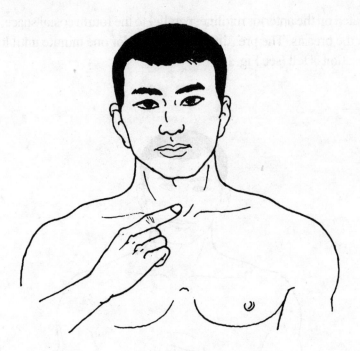

Fig. 2 Pressing Tiantu

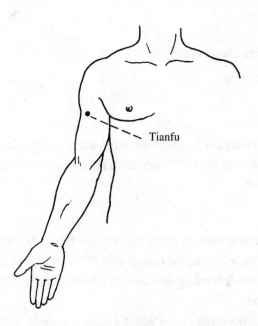

Fig. 3 Tianfu

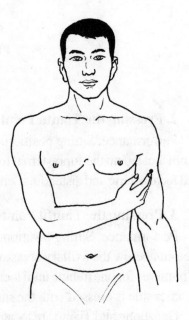

Fig. 4 Pressing Tianfu

4. Stroking the Neck and Nape

Performance: Sitting position. The palms and fingers of both hands are used during the performance. First, the palm and four fingers of one hand are used to stroke the neck from the clavicle, along the earlobe and to the cervical vertebrae continuously for about one minute until the area feels warm (see Fig. 5). Then the other side is rubbed the same way.

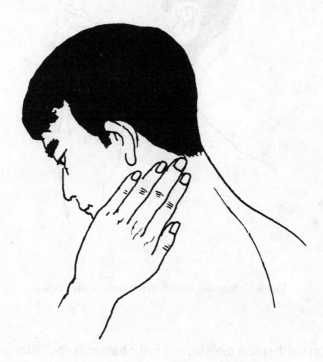

Fig. 5 Stroking the neck and nape

5. Rubbing the Front of the Neck

Performance: Sitting position. The thumb and four fingers of both hands are used alternatively during the performance. First, the thumb and four fingers of one hand rub the sides of the larynx upward and downward for about one minute until a local warm sensation is felt (see Fig. 6). Then the other side is done with the same method.

The neck supports the head and is connected to the trunk of the body. The governor vessel flows through the center of the neck. The bladder meridian flows along the sides of the neck; the triple energizer meridian flows beside the bladder meridian and behind the ears; the gallbladder meridian flows below the ears; and the large intestine meridian, small intestine meridian and the stomach meridian flow along the sides of the larynx. The neck is the passage

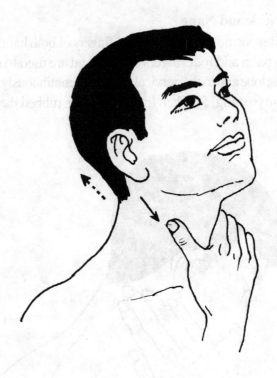

Fig. 6 Massaging the anterior part of the neck

of the throat and is one of the most mobile parts in the human body. So this method is effective in smoothing the joints, eliminating pathogenic wind, dredging meridians, activating collaterals, promoting digestion and removing stagnation.

6. Pushing and Kneading the Chest

① Performance: Sitting position. The palms and the fingers of both hands are used to push and knead from the upper part to the lower part of the sternum on the opposite side and then along the sternum sides to the shoulder and armpit. The pushing and kneading are done continuously for one minute until a local warm sensation is felt and breathing becomes regular (see Fig. 7). Then the other side is pushed and kneaded the same way.

② Effect: This method can disperse stagnant pulmonary *qi*, and relieve superficial pathogenic factors as it soothes the chest and regulates *qi*.

7. Squeezing the Upper Part of the Back

① Performance: Sitting position. The palms and fingers of both hands are used to squeeze-release continuously from the nape to the upper part of the back for about one minute (see Fig. 8) until a local warm sensation is felt. The right hand works first, then the left hand.

② Effect: This technique can relax the tendons, relieve spasms and stop pain.

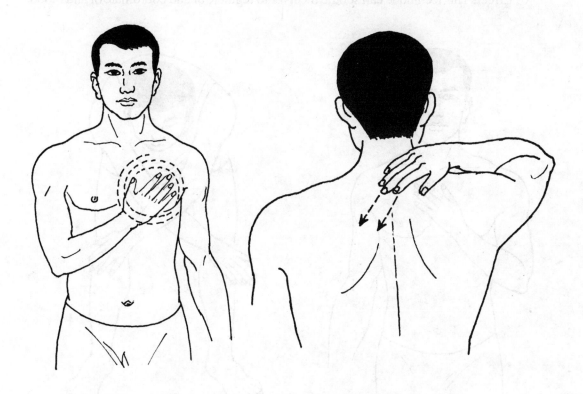

| Fig. 7 Pushing and kneading chest | Fig. 8 Squeezing the upper part of the back |

8. Patting the Chest

① Performance: Sitting position with body relaxed. The fingers of both hands are slightly bent and held together. The hands are used alternatively to pat the chest from the sternum border, along the intercostal space to the region below the armpit and shoulder. The patting is done repeatedly for about two minutes (see Fig. 9).

② Effect: This performance can sooth the chest to regulate *qi* and loosen phlegm to relieve asthma.

9. Bending at the Waist to Exhale *Qi*

① Performance: Sitting position with body relaxed, breathing through the nose, and without any thought of straining. The forearms are crossed over the abdomen and the body is bent to exhale (see Fig. 10). It is necessary to exhale as deep as possible. Then slowly sit up, gradually raise the arms and inhale. This performance is done continuously for about two minutes.

② Effect: This technique can soothe the liver to regulate *qi* and coordinate *qi* and blood.

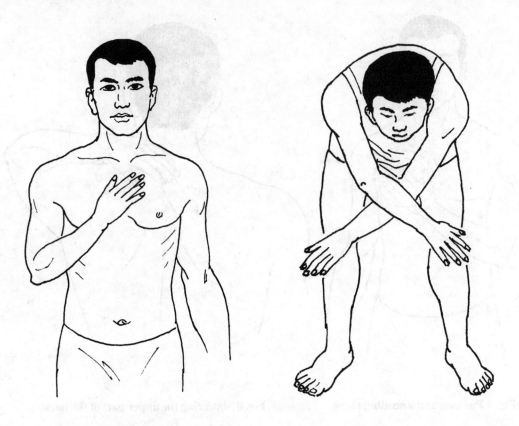

Fig. 9 Patting the chest   **Fig. 10 Bending at the waist to exhale**

Notes:

1. When asthma is in remission, self-massage along meridians and acupoints is done one to two times a day in combination with prescribed drugs and physical exercise, which helps to shorten the therapeutic course of asthma while preventing relapses and prolonging intervals between attacks.

2. Care should be taken to avoid inhaling allergic factors and to wear clothing appropriate to the season to avoid catching a common cold.

3. Keep in a cheerful frame of mind, take light food and avoid tobacco and alcoholic beverages.

Section 4 Coronary Heart Disease

Introduction

Coronary heart disease, also known as ischemic heart disease, is commonly seen among the middle-aged and elderly. The coronary vessel is the main artery connected with the heart, the route through which blood is supplied to the heart to nourish the myocardium. Atheromatous sclerosis occurs in the coronary artery when cholesterol begins to line the wall of the coronary artery, leading to a constriction of the artery which in turn results in the reduction of the myocardial supply of blood. The resulting insufficient supply of oxygen can lead to chest pains or even a heart attack.

The cause of coronary heart disease is generally considered to be prolonged excessive intake of calories and fat, especially an excessive intake of foods high in saturated fats and cholesterol. Diabetes and hypertension also frequently lead to coronary heart disease.

Traditional Chinese medicine holds that "blood serves to moisten the body and *qi* serves to warm the body." The viscera depend on blood to moisten and nourish, while blood depends on *qi* to promote circulation. Any impairment of this internal balance by excessive emotion (joy, anger, anxiety, worry, sadness, fear and fright), improper diet, cold pathogenic factors and asthenia of kidney *qi* may result in stagnation of *qi* and stasis of blood which consequently leads to coronary heart disease.

The Main Symptoms of Coronary Heart Disease

Latent coronary heart disease, often seen among people middle-aged or older, is marked by atheromatous sclerosis in the coronary artery without noticeable symptoms, but with obvious or constant elevation of the cholesterol index in the blood and the possibility of myocardiac ischemia shown in electrocardiograph tests.

Angina pectoris is characterized by a pressing or squeezing pain in the precardium, behind the sternum or in the deep region of the anterior part of the thorax that may radiate to the left shoulder and arm. The attack may last for two to three minutes. It is usually induced by overstrain, cold, excessive eating and excitement. Usually it can be relieved by resting or taking nitroglycerin tablets.

Myocardial infarction is marked by pain behind the sternum or in the precardium accompanied by a contracting or squeezing sensation. In serious cases, the pain is sharp, prolonged and radiates to the neck, shoulder and arm. The patient usually manifests restlessness; cold limbs; thin, weak and rapid pulse; even lowering of blood pressure, coma, heart failure and arrhythmia. An electrocardiograph shows obvious changes of S-T section and T wave.

Manipulations for Self-Massage Along Meridians and Acupoints

1. Pressing the Fengfu Point (GV 16)

Performance: Sitting position. The tip of the thumb of one hand is placed on the vertex with the rest four fingers naturally bent. The thumb, placed on Fengfu located 0.5 *cun* directly over the median point of the posterior hairline, presses and massages repeatedly for one minute until local distending and comfortable sensation is felt (see Fig. 1).

Fengfu is a confluent acupoint of the Governor Vessel, Bladder Meridian and Yangwei Vessel. Deep inside the Fengfu pass the vertebral artery, occipital artery and occipital nerve. This area is the key region for treating coronary heart disease by means of self-massage along meridians and acupoints.

2. Pressing the Bulang Point (KI 22)

Performance: Sitting position. Both tips of the thumbs are placed on Bulang, located on the fifth inter-costal space and two *cun* lateral to the anterior midline, and press repeatedly for one minute until a local distending and comfortable sensation is felt (see Fig. 2). Then the hands are exchanged to press the opposite sides.

3. Pressing the Ximen Point (PC 4)

Performance: Sitting position. Both tips of the thumbs are placed alternately on Ximen located 5 *cun* directly above the median point of the wrist crease and between the two tendons, and press repeatedly for one minute until a local aching, distending, numb and electrical sensation radiated to the tips of the fingers is felt (see Fig. 3). Then the hands are exchanged to press the opposite side with the same method.

4. Pressing the Neiguan Point (PC 6)

Performance: Sitting position. The tips of thumbs are placed on Neiguan, located two *cun* directly above the median point of the wrist crease and between the two tendons, and press repeatedly for one minute until a local numb and distending sensation is felt radiating to the elbow, armpit and chest (see Fig. 4). Then the hands are exchanged to press the opposite side with the same method.

Fengfu is located on the Governor Vessel, Bulang on the kidney meridian, Ximen

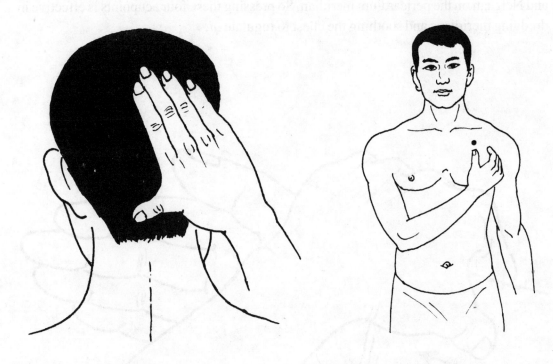

Fig. 1 Pressing Fengfu

Fig. 2 Pressing Bulang

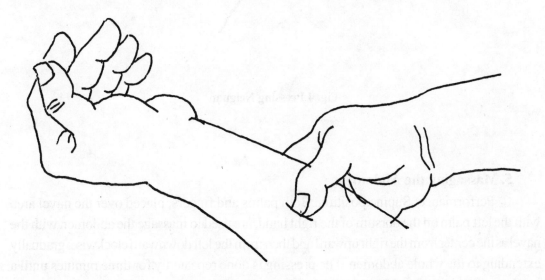

Fig. 3 Pressing Ximen

and Neiguan on the pericardium meridian. So pressing these four acupoints is effective in dredging meridians and soothing the chest to regulate *qi*.

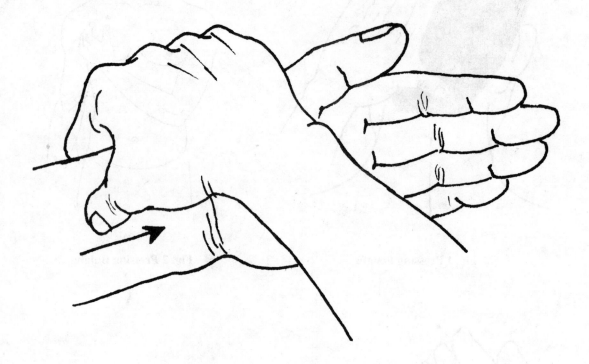

Fig. 4 Pressing Neiguan

5. Massaging the Abdomen

① Performance: Supine position. Both palms and fingers, placed over the navel area with the left palm on the dorsum of the right hand, are used to massage the abdomen with the navel as the center from the right upward and then from the left downward clockwise, gradually extending to the whole abdomen. The pressing is done repeatedly for three minutes until a local warm and comfortable sensation is felt (see Fig. 5).

② Effect: This technique may dredge meridians.

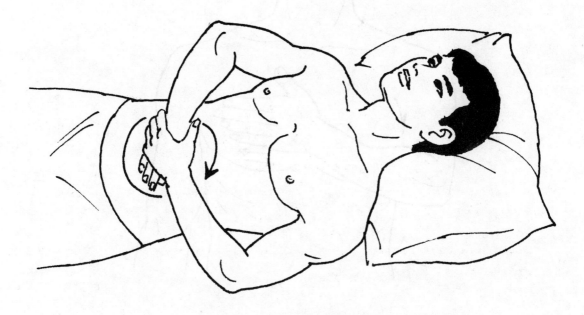

Fig. 5 Massaging abdomen

6. Pushing and Pressing the Chest

① Performance: Sitting position. Both palms and fingers are used alternatively to press. The right hand is used to press first from upper part of the sternum to the lower part on the left. The pressing is also done along both sides of the sternum to the shoulder and armpit repeatedly for about one minute until a local warm and comfortable sensation is felt (see Fig. 6). Then the left hand is used to press the right side with the same method.

② Effect: This performance can remove retention and eliminate stagnation as well as regulate *qi* and relieve pain.

7. Squeezing and Holding the Upper Part of the Back

① Performance: Sitting position. Both palms and fingers are used alternatively to press. The right palm is placed on the upper part of the back and squeezes from the upper to the lower and from the left shoulder to the right shoulder repeatedly for about one minute (see Fig. 7 ① ②) until a local warm and comfortable sensation is felt. Then the left hand is used to pinch with the same method.

② Effect: This method is effective in relieving spasm and pain.

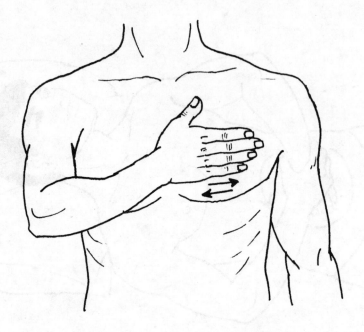

Fig. 6 Pushing and pressing chest

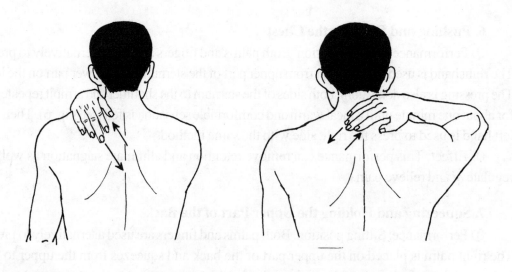

① Squeezing the upper part of the back on the opposite side

② Squeezing the upper part of the back on the same side

Fig. 7 Squeezing and holding the upper part of the back

8. Patting the Chest

① Performance: Sitting position. The fingers of both hands are closed and slightly bent. One hand is used to pat the opposite side of the chest from the border of the sternum, along the inter-costal space to the shoulder and armpit repeatedly for about one minute (see Fig. 8). Then the other hand is used to pat the opposite side of the chest using the same method.

② Effect: This method can soothe the chest, regulate *qi*, eliminate retention and resolve stagnation.

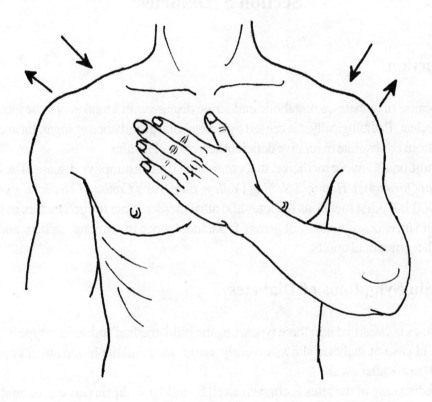

Fig. 8 Patting the chest

Notes:

1. It has been shown that long-term application of self-massage along meridians and acupoints (in the morning and evening every day) before or after the onset of coronary heart disease can both prevent and treat coronary heart disease. Self-massage along meridians and

acupoints is good for regulating the functions of the heart, alleviating spasms of the coronary artery and improving myocardial ischemia.

2. Keep in a good mood, follow a vegetarian diet, avoid smoking and restrict drinking.

3. Alternate work with rest and recreation, avoid being attacked by cold.

4. Participate in suitable physical activities, such as *qigong* (or breathing exercise) and *Taijiquan* (or Taiji boxing), etc.

Section 5 Diabetes

Introduction

The cause of diabetes, a metabolic endocrine disease with a tendency to be inherited, is usually unclear. Pathologically it is caused by a metabolic disturbance of sugar, fat and protein resulting from an absolute or relative deficient secretion of insulin.

In traditional Chinese medicine, diabetes is called a consumptive disease. The book *Su Wen (Plain Questions). Huangdi Neijing (Yellow Emperor's Canon of Medicine),* compiled in about 400 B.C, first mentions diabetes and attributes its cause to such factors as frequent asthenia of *yin,* excessive eating of greasy food, indulgence in drinking, anxiety and rage as well as other emotional upsets.

The Main Symptoms of Diabetes

Diabetes is classified into three types, i.e., the mild, median and serious types:

A mild case of diabetes shows no early symptoms, and the blood sugar is probably below 150 mg% after meal.

A median case of diabetes is characterized by mild polydipsia (excessive or abnormal thirst), polyphagia (excessive desire to eat), polyuria (excessive need to urinate), emaciation, headache, pain in the legs, insomnia, hypopsia (diminution of vision) and irregular menstruation. In the male, a decline in sexual interest may occur. The occurrence of high urine sugar is usually accompanied by blood sugar.

The serious type of diabetes may occur before the age of 15. Usually the onset is prolonged. Apart from the appearance of urine sugar and the increase of blood sugar from the symptoms mentioned above, there are secondary symptoms, the usual ones of which are acute infection, pulmonary tuberculosis, hypertension and arteriosclerosis. The blood sugar is usually over 250 mg% on an empty stomach. In serious cases, there may appear ketoacidosis (insulin deficiency) and diabetic coma.

Application of Self-Massage Along Meridians and Acupoints

1. Rubbing the Face

Performance: Sitting position. Both palms and fingers are rubbed warm and then are used to rub the face in the area from the lips to the sides of the nose, around the eyes, forehead and ears like washing the face. The rubbing continues for about two minutes until a warm sensation is felt all over the face (see Fig. 1).

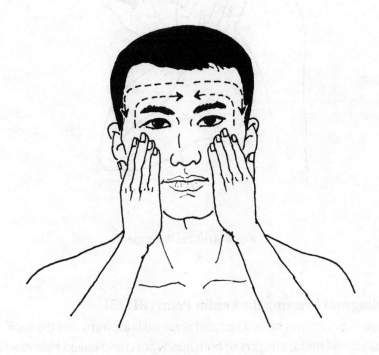

Fig. 1 Rubbing the face

2. Stroking the Nape

Performance: Sitting position. The fingers of both hands intertwine and then embrace the nape. The head is slightly raised backward and then both hands stroke the nape in as wide a range as possible for about one minute (see Fig. 2).

The massage should be done in a moderate and gentle way. The eyes are closed and the mind is calm, keeping in good mood and breathing naturally.

The two methods mentioned above are effective in tranquilizing the mind, refreshing the brain and improving eyesight.

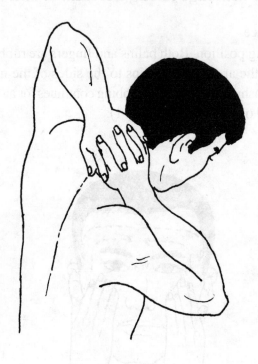

Fig. 2 Stroking the nape

3. Kneading and Pressing the Feishu Point (BL 13)

Performance: Sitting position. The head is raised backward and the back and waist are relaxed. The index and middle fingers of both hands press and knead Feishu which is 1.5 *cun* inferior and lateral to the third thoracic vertebral process for about one minute. The application is light at first and then becomes heavier until a local aching and distending sensation is felt (see Fig. 3).

4. Pressing and Kneading the Weishu (BL 21) and Shenshu Points (BL 23)

Performance: Sitting position and relaxation of the waist and back. Both hands form into fists, the knuckles are used to press and knead Weishu 1.5 *cun* inferior and lateral to the 12th thoracic vertebral process and Shenshu inferior and lateral to the second lumbar vertebral process for about three minutes. The application is light at first and then becomes heavier until a local aching and distending sensation is felt (see Fig. 4).

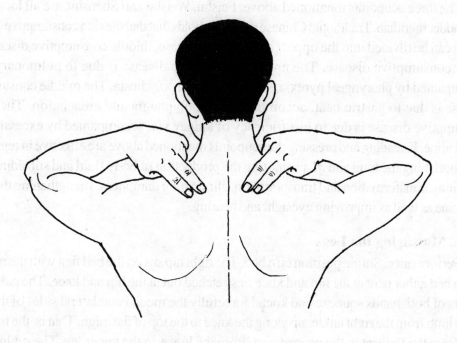

Fig. 3 Pressing and kneading Feishu

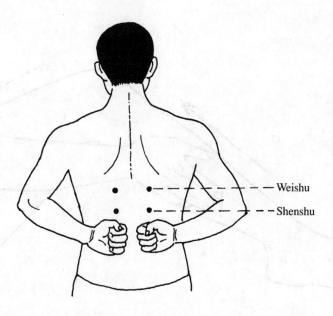

Weishu

Shenshu

Fig. 4 Pressing and kneading Weishu and Shenshu

The three acupoints mentioned above, Feishu, Weishu and Shenshu, are all located on the bladder meridian. Traditional Chinese medicine holds that diabetes is a consumptive disease which can be divided into the upper consumptive disease, middle consumptive disease and lower consumptive disease. The upper consumptive disease is due to pulmonary heat, accompanied by pharyngeal pyrexia, severe thirst and polydipsia. The middle consumptive disease is due to gastric heat, accompanied by polyphagia and emaciation. The lower consumptive disease is due to insufficiency of kidney *yin*, accompanied by excessive and turbid urine. Kneading and pressing the acupoints mentioned above are effective in regulating and nourishing the lung and *qi*, promoting the production of body fluid and subsiding heat, benefiting transformation and transportation, eliminating dampness, strengthening the waist and spine as well as improving eyesight and hearing.

5. Massaging the Legs

Performance: Sitting position on a bed. The right hip sits on the bed first with the right leg on the bed either bent at the hip and knee or stretched out at the hip and knee. The palms and fingers of both hands squeeze and knead forcefully the medial and lateral sides of the right lower limb from the right ankle, up along the knee to the top of the thigh. That is, the massage goes from the farthest to the nearest part, from the lower to the upper leg. The rubbing and kneading are done all around the leg and repeatedly for three minutes (see Fig. 5). Then the left hip sits on the bed, and both hands massage the left leg in the same way.

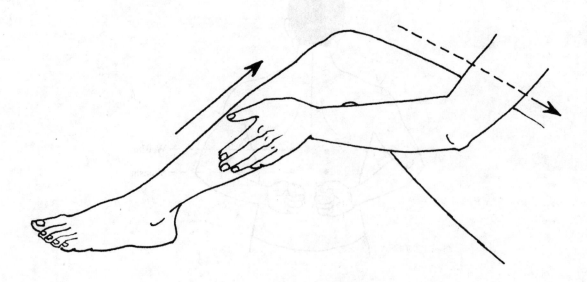

Fig. 5 Massaging the legs

6. Massaging the Arms

Performance: Sitting position. The right palm and fingers squeeze and knead the left arm from the wrist, up along the elbow to the shoulder. The massage is done all around the arm and repeatedly from the lateral to the medial side and from the lower to the upper for two minutes (see Fig. 6). Then the left hand massages the right arm in the same way.

Notes:

1. The massage should be heavy enough to produce stimulating effects and moderate enough to avoid injury of the muscle, vessel and skin.

2. The above two methods are effective in improving blood and lymph circulation, promoting metabolism and strengthening the muscles.

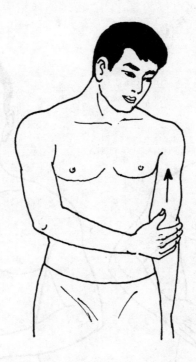

Fig. 6 Massaging the arms

7. Pushing and Pressing the Lower Abdomen

Performance: Supination. The hips and knees are bent, the abdomen is relaxed and the respiration is natural.

The palms and fingers of both hands are placed on the sides of the abdomen, pushing the abdominal wall from the upper to the lower for about two minutes (see Fig. 7) to relax abdominal tension.

8. Pressing and Kneading the Abdomen

Performance: Supination. The hips and knee are bent, the abdomen is relaxed and the respiration is natural.

The palm of the left hand is placed on the back of the right hand over the navel. Both hands press and knead the abdomen clockwise from the right to the upper and from the left to the lower repeatedly for about five minutes. The massage is light at first and then heavier until a warm and comfortable sensation is felt inside the abdomen (see Fig. 8).

The above two methods are effective in dredging meridians, promoting metabolism and regulating the functions of the viscera. They are the basic techniques used to treat diabetes.

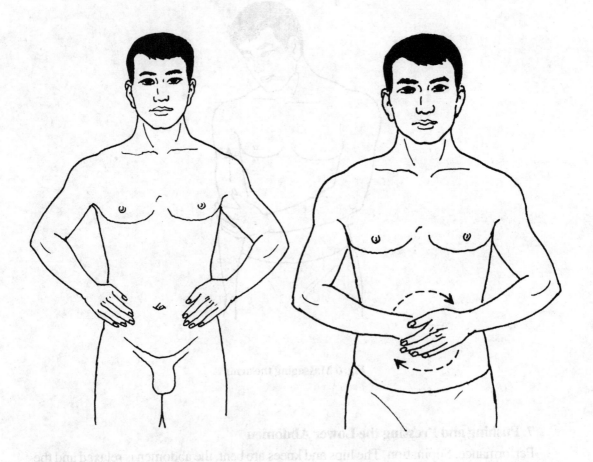

Fig. 7 Pushing and pressing lower abdomen   Fig. 8 Pressing and kneading abdomen

Notes:

1. Diabetes is a chronic disease, requiring a longer course of treatment. So the patient should have confidence and keep performing self-massage along meridians and acupoints in the morning and evening. This manipulation is effective in treating diabetes of mild and median types. If the symptoms are already serious with high blood sugar level and high urine sugar, diabetes should be treated with drugs.

2. The diet must be restricted. Reasonable amounts of vegetables, soybeans, lean meats and eggs can be enjoyed. Greasy and rich foods should be avoided.

3. Get proper physical exercise but avoid overstraining.

4. Keep in good mood, maintain regular daily activities and avoid mental stress.

Section 6 Hypertension

Introduction

Hypertension is a chronic disease mainly caused by a disturbance of cerebral cortical functions and vascular diastolization and contraction. Etiologically symptomatic hypertension is excluded. The main clinical manifestation is an increase of blood pressure in the artery. The complications in the advanced stage are acute cerebral vascular disease and hypertensive heart disease, etc.

In traditional Chinese medicine, hypertension is generally believed to be caused by a disorder of the liver and kidney meridians, asthenia of liver and kidney *yin* and hyperactivity of liver *yang* as well as an imbalance between *yin* and *yang*.

The Symptoms of Hypertension

Hypertension is marked by continuous lingering over 140/90 mmHg (in the mercury column), accompanied at the same time by vertigo, headache, distension of the head, tinnitus, blurred vision, insomnia, palpitations, numbness of the fingers, chest distress, restlessness and apathy. In serious cases the symptoms may be aggravated and the blood pressure may rapidly increase, usually accompanied by such symptoms as asevere headache, angina pectoris, dyspnea, even nausea, vomiting and coma.

Application of Self-Massage Along Meridians and Acupoints

1. Massaging the Renying Point (ST 9)

① Performance: Sitting. The head leans slightly to the right side. The thumb of the right hand is slightly bent and the fingers, held together, massage around Renying (located on the side of the neck, parallel to the Adam's apple, at the cervical artery and the anterior border of the sternocleidomastoid muscle) from the posterior border of the ear lobe toward the chest. The massaging is done repeatedly for about one minute (see Fig. 2).

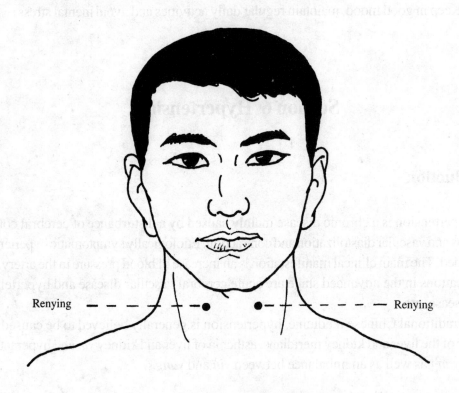

Renying —————————————————— Renying

Fig. 1 Renying

Then the head leans slightly to the left, and the left hand massages Renying on the right side in the same way.

Renying should not be massaged on both sides at the same time. The massage should be done on one side first, and then the other. Care should be taken to avoid over-massaging both in pressure and time. When a masseur is doing the technique, the patient may be asked to

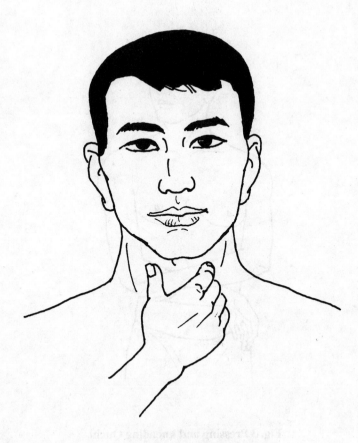

Fig. 2 Massaging Renying

move the head and neck simultaneously.

② Effect: This method can help relieve symptoms and lower blood pressure.

2. Pressing and Kneading the Quchi Point (LI 11)

① Performance: Sitting position. The right thumb is used to press right Quchi (located in the depression lateral to the elbow crease when the elbow is bent) for three minutes until a local aching and distending sensation radiates to the forearm (see Fig. 3).

Then the left thumb is used to press Quchi on the right side in the same way.

② Effect: Quchi is located on the large intestine meridian. This method is effective in regulating *qi* and blood and lowering blood pressure.

3. Stroking the Yongquan Point (KI 1)

① Performance: Sitting position. The right foot is placed on the left knee. The right hand

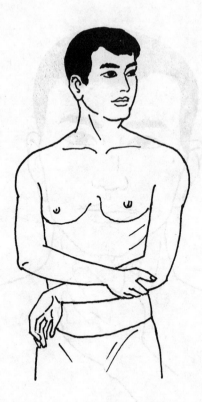

Fig. 3 Pressing and kneading Quchi

grasps the right foot and the left palm is used to stroke Yongquan (located on the point 1/3 anterior and 2/3 posterior to the center of the sole) for about three minutes until a local warm, aching and distending sensation is felt (see Fig. 4).

Then the left foot is placed on the right knee, the left hand grasps the left foot and the right palm strokes Yongquan on the left foot in the same way.

② Effect: Yongquan is located on the kidney meridian. This method of using Laogong (PC 8) in the center of the palm to stroke Yongquan is effective in tranquilizing and lowering blood pressure.

4. Pressing the Fengchi Point (GB 20)

① Performance: Sitting position. The thumbs of both hands are placed over Fengchi (located in the depression between the sternocleidomastoid muscle and trapezius muscle) with the fingers fixed on the occipital region. The thumbs are used to press Fengchi for about three minutes until a local aching and distending sensation is felt (see Fig. 5).

(6) Effect: Tension School—Liu, the Gallbladder meridian. So this method is effective in dispelling wind and relieving superficial pain caused by exogenous wind and in activating the brain and improving eyesight.

3. Massaging the Abdomen

① Performance: Supination with hips and abdomen relaxed and the knees bent. The right palm is placed over the navel and the left hand rests upon the right hand. Both hands press down to and fro in a circular motion starting with a small range recover the whole abdomen location to strengthen self-awareness to comfort the sensation of the conditions the navel area of abdomen. (see Fig. 3)

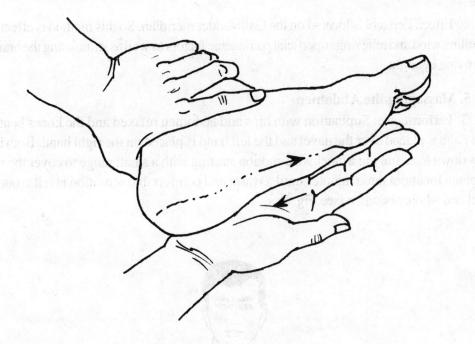

Fig. 4 Stroking Yongquan

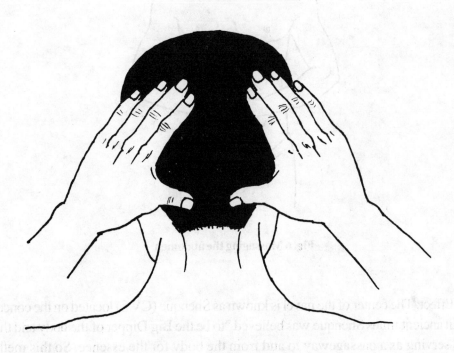

Fig. 5 Pressing Fengchi

② Effect: Fengchi is located on the Gallbladder meridian. So this method is effective in dispelling wind and relieving superficial pathogenic factors as well as stimulating the brain and improving eyesight.

5. Massaging the Abdomen

① Performance: Supination with hips and abdomen relaxed and the knees bent. The right palm is placed over the navel and the left hand is placed on the right hand. Both hands press down forcefully in a clockwise-motion starting with a small range to cover the whole abdomen for about three minutes until a warm and comfortable sensation is felt around the navel and whole abdomen (see Fig. 6).

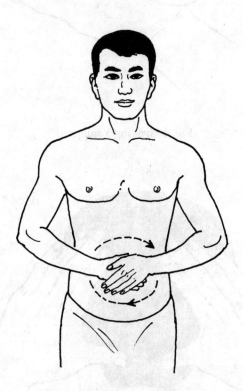

Fig. 6 Massaging the abdomen

② Effect: The center of the navel is known as Shenque (CV 8) located on the conception vessel. In ancient times Shenque was believed "to be the Big Dipper of the body and the root of life," serving as a passageway to and from the body for the essence. So this method is effective in communicating with the meridians, regulating the conditions of *yin* and *yang* as well as lowering blood pressure.

Notes:

1. Self-massage along meridians and acupoints should be done frequently, usually one or two times a day. It is significantly effective in treating patients with mild symptoms who have had hypertension for a short time.

2. Daily activities must be regular, and proper physical exercise is required.

3. Avoid mental tension and overstrain and keep optimistic.

4. Avoid smoking and alcohol; follow a vegetarian diet and eat moderately.

Section 7 Impotence

Introduction

Impotence refers to inability of the penis to erect or fully erect, despite a desire for sexual intercourse. Impotence, except in a few organic pathological instances (such as deformity or maldevelopment of the genitals, chronic inflammation, chronic prostatitis, hypogenesis of the testicles and mental illness) is mainly a problem of function caused by mental tension, over-excitement, or fear, rage, anxiety, excessive sexual activity and masturbation.

Traditional Chinese medicine holds that impotence is usually caused by excessive sexual activity, or masturbation, or anxiety, or timidity, susceptibility to fright and terror, which eventually impairs the kidney. Since the kidney governs reproduction, the impairment of the kidney may lead to impotence. It may also be caused by a congenital weakness of the body or weakness due to prolonged illness. So the treatment of impotence should focus on the primary causes, avoiding misusing tonics warm in nature.

Symptoms of Impotence

The usual symptoms are a lack of interest in sex and the inability of the penis to erect or fully erect during sexual intercourse, often accompanied by vertigo, dizziness, insomnia, lethargy and aching and weakness in the waist and knees. After any overstraining or drinking to excess, occasional impotence is not considered serious. Only long term and frequent impotence is regarded as a health problem.

Manipulations for Self-Massage Along Meridians and Acupoints

1. Pressing the Qihai (CV 6) and Guanyuan Points (CV 4)

Performance: Supination with the abdomen relaxed and the knees and hips bent. The tip of the middle finger of one hand is used to press Qihai (located 1.5 *cun* directly below the center of the navel) and Guanyuan (located three *cun* directly below the center of the navel) for two minutes each (see Fig. 1).

The massage should be gentle, appropriate and penetrating until a local aching and distending sensation radiates to the penis.

2. Pressing the Shenshu Point (BL 23)

Performance: Sitting position with the relaxation of the waist and back. Both hands form into fists to press Shenshu (located 1.5 *cun* inferior and lateral to the second lumbar vertebral process) for about two minutes (see Fig. 2).

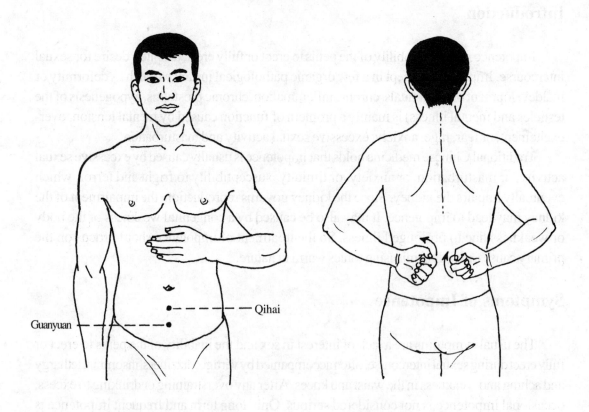

Fig. 1 Pressing acupoints   **Fig. 2 Pressing Shenshu**

3. Pressing the Sanyinjiao Point (SP 6)

Performance: Sitting position. The right lower leg is placed on the upper part of the left knee and the left hand grasps the right ankle. The right thumb presses Sanyinjiao (located three *cun* directly above the tip of the medial ankle) for about one minute until a local aching and distending sensation is felt (see Fig. 3). Then Sanyinjiao on the left foot is pressed in the same way.

Qihai and Guanyuan are the acupoints located on the conception vessel and are the key acupoints selected to treat impotence. Shenshu is located on the bladder meridian and Sanyinjiao is on the spleen meridian. This method is effective in strengthening the kidney to consolidate the base of life and soothing the liver to eliminate stagnation.

4. Pushing and Kneading the Lower Abdomen

① Performance: Supination with a relaxed abdomen and knees bent. Both palms and fingers are used to push and knead the lower abdomen from the navel to the groin for about three minutes (see Fig. 4).

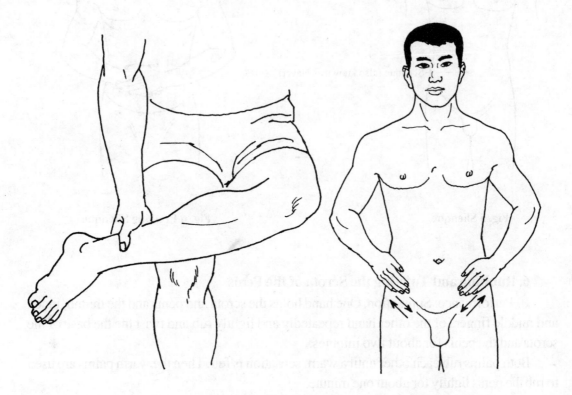

Fig. 3 Pressing Sanyinjiao   Fig. 4 Pushing and kneading the lower abdomen

② Effect: This technique can help dredge meridians and eliminate damp-heat.

5. Pressing the Shenque Point (CV 8)

① Performance: Supination with hip and knees bent. The right palm is placed on the navel (see Fig. 5), and the left hand is placed over the right hand. Both hands press and rotate over the navel for about two minutes (see Fig. 6).

② Effect: Shenque is located on the conception vessel. So this method is effective in invigorating the spleen and stomach as well as in warming and dredging the meridians.

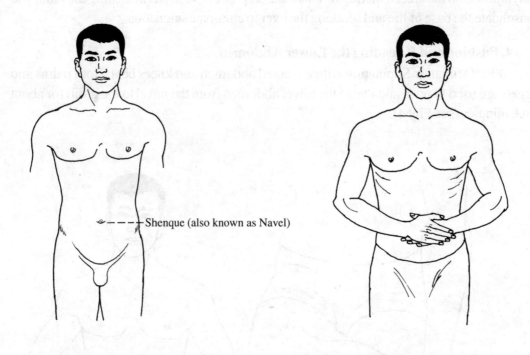

Shenque (also known as Navel)

Fig. 5 Shenque   **Fig. 6 Pressing Shenque**

6. Rubbing and Twisting the Scrota of the Penis

① Performance: Supination. One hand holds the scrota and penis and the thumb, index and middle fingers of the other hand repeatedly and lightly rub and twist the the base of the scrota and the penis for about two minutes.

Both palms rub each other until a warm sensation is felt. Then the warm palms are used to rub the penis lightly for about one minute.

Note: The rubbing should be done gently. If the penis has an erection, the rubbing can be continued until a slight local distending sensation is felt. When rubbing and twisting the scrota and penis, the patient should repeatedly contract the anus and the lower abdomen for about half a minute.

② Effect: This method is effective in regulating *qi* and restoreing *yang*.

7. Stroking the Lumbosacral Region

① Performance: Sitting position with a slight bending at the waist. The fingers of both hands are closed and are placed against the lumbosacral region to stroke from the upper to the lower for about two minutes until the skin turns reddish and a warm sensation is felt (see Fig. 7).

② Effect: It can strengthen the waist and invigorate the kidney.

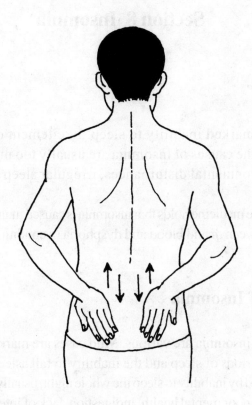

Fig. 7 Stroking the lumbosacral region

Notes:

1. Self-massage along meridians and acupoints should be done once every night before

sleep. This method is especially effective in treating functional impotence due to psychological factors.

2. The patient should have confidence that his impotence can be cured. Care from the wife is also very important. During treatment, sexual intercourse should be replaced by caressing and kissing. It is best for the couple to sleep separately.

3. Attempts should be made to do regular physical exercise to strengthen the body and steady the mind. A balance should be maintained between work and leisure.

4. Sexual intercourse should be restricted until impotence is cured.

Section 8 Insomnia

Introduction

Insomnia is the marked inability to sleep. Excitement or anxiety may make it difficult to sleep. So the causes of insomnia are usually too much thinking, too much mental tension, environmental disturbances, irregular sleep patterns, neurasthenia, menopause, etc.

Traditional Chinese medicine holds that insomnia is caused mainly by a dysfunction of the viscera, imbalance between *qi* and blood and dysphoria (a condition marked by anxiety and despondency).

The Symptoms of Insomnia

The symptoms of insomnia are various. Mild cases are marked by difficulty in sleep, shallow sleep, short periods of sleep and the inability to fall asleep again after waking up. Serious cases are marked by inability to sleep the whole night, usually accompanied by vertigo, headache, palpitations, poor mental health, indigestion, lack of interest in eating, fatigue and poor memory, etc.

Manipulations for Self-Massage Along Meridians and Acupoints

1. Pressing the Fengchi Point (GB 20)
Performance: Sitting position. The thumbs of both hands press on Fenchi (located in the

depression below the occipital bone, parallel to the lower border of the mastoid process and lateral to the large tendon) and the fingers are fixed on the posterior part of the occipital bone. The pressing is done repeatedly for about a minute (see Fig. 1).

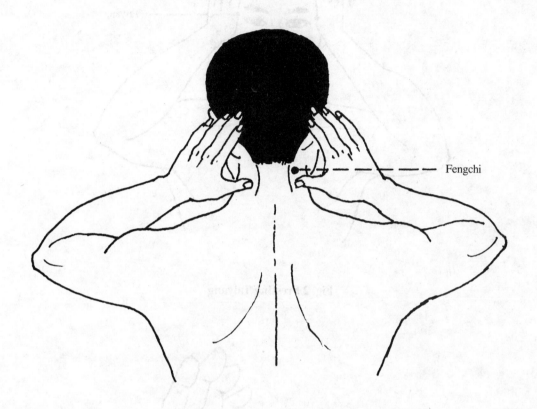

Fig. 1 Pressing Fengchi

2. Pressing Taiyang (EX-HN 5)

Performance: Sitting position. Both hands are used to press Taiyang (located on the temporal side and in the depression on the median point of the line connecting the end of the eyebrow with the outer canthus). The pressing is done repeatedly for about a minute (see Fig. 2).

3. Pressing Shenmen (HT 7)

Performance: Sitting position. Both hands are used alternatively to press Shenmen (located in the depression slight superior to the ulnar side of the crease on the wrist) of both hands for a minute each.

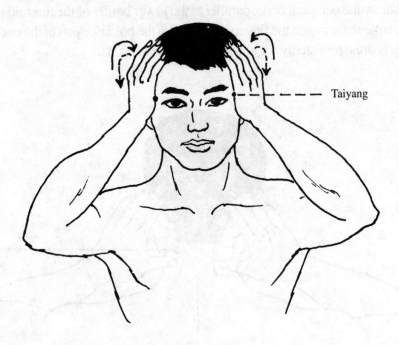

Fig. 2 Pressing Taiyang

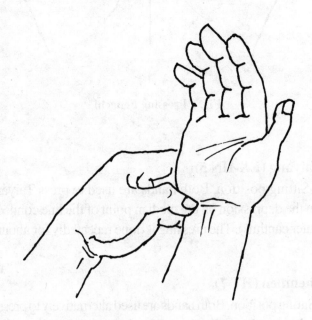

Fig. 3 Pressing Shenmen

4. Pressing Sanyinjiao (SP 6)

Performance: Sitting position. The thumb is used alternatively to press Sanyinjiao (located three *cun* directly above the tip of the medial ankle and on the posterior border of the tibia) for one minute on each leg (see Fig. 4).

The above acupoints are pressed until a local aching and distending sensation is felt. Fengchi is located on the gallbladder meridian, Taiyang on the extraordinary meridian, Shenmen on the heart meridian and Sanyinjiao on the spleen meridian. This massage is effective in tranquilizing the mind and eliminating stagnation as well as regulating *qi* and blood.

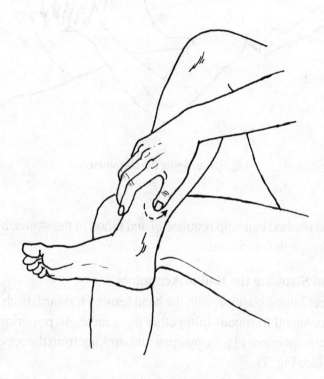

Fig. 4 Pressing Sanyinjiao

5. Massaging the Abdomen

① Performance: Supination with hips and knees bent and abdomen relaxed. The right hand is placed on the upper abdomen and the left hand is placed over the right hand. Both hands press and massage the abdomen from the upper part to the lower part along the midline of the abdomen for about two minutes (see Fig. 5).

The massage should be swift and gentle, mild at first and then heavier until a warm sensation is felt in the abdomen.

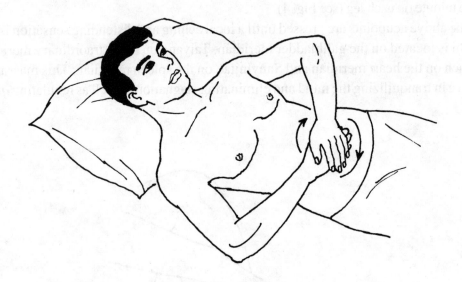

Fig. 5 Massaging the abdomen

② Effect: This method can help regulate *qi* and blood in the stomach and intestines as well as warm and dredge the meridians.

6. Pushing and Stroking the Baliao Acupoints

① Performance: Sitting position with the head leaning forward. Both hands are placed on the four posterior sacral foramens (altogether there are eight posterior sacral foramens known as Baliao acupoints) (see Fig. 6), pushing and stroking from the upper to the lower for about two minutes (see Fig. 7).

② Effect: Baliao acupoints are located on the bladder meridian. This method is effective in strengthening the waist and supplementing the kidney as well as regulating *qi* and blood.

7. Stroking the Yongquan Point (KI 1)

① Performance: Sitting position. The right foot is placed on the left knee and the right hand grasps the right foot. The ulnar side (side opposite the thumb) of the left palm is placed on Yongquan (located on the point 1/3 anterior to and 2/3 posterior to the midline of the sole) and strokes for three minutes until a local warm, aching and distending sensation is felt (see Fig. 9).

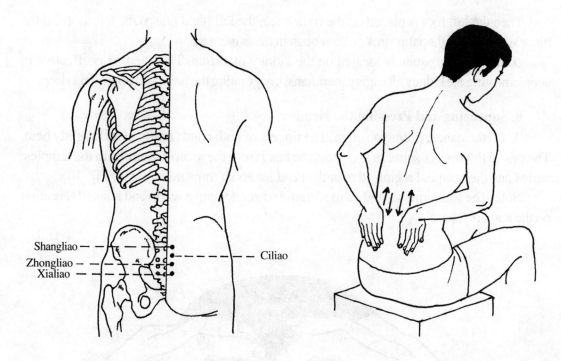

Fig.6 Baliao (posterior sacral foramens)

Shangliao
Zhongliao
Xialiao
Ciliao

Fig. 7 Pushing and stroking Baliao

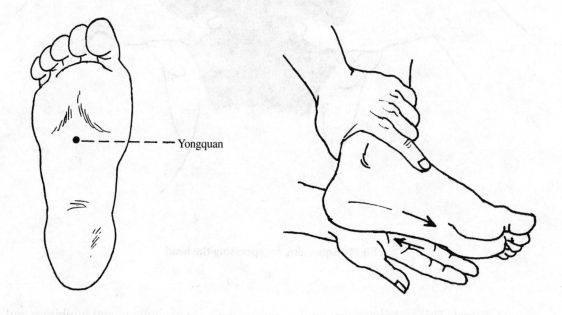

Yongquan

Fig. 8 Yongquan

Fig. 9 Stroking Yongquan

Then the left foot is placed on the right knee, the left hand grasps the left foot and the ulnar side of the right palm strokes Yongquan in the same way.

② Effect: Yongquan is located on the kidney meridian. This method is effective in supplementing the kidney, dredging meridians, invigorating the brain and improving sleep.

8. Squeezing and Pressing the Head

① Performance: Sitting position. The fingers of both hands are open and slightly bent. The tips of the fingers squeeze and press the head from the anterior hairline to the temples, vertex and the occipital region all over the head for about three minutes (see Fig. 10).

Note: The technique should be moderate and gentle until a warm and relaxed sensation on the scalp is felt.

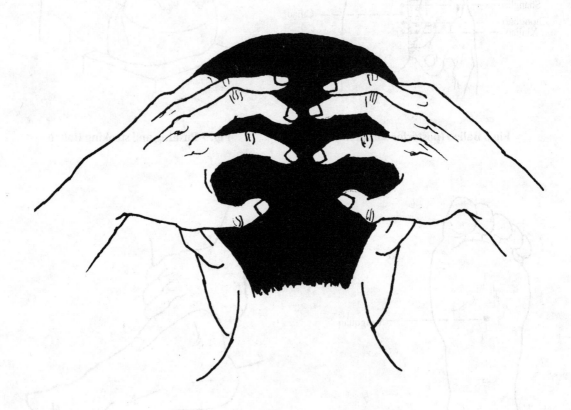

Fig. 10 Squeezing and pressing the head

② Effect: This technique can regulate nerves, balance excitement and inhibition and relax the over-taxed brain so as to cure insomnia.

Notes:

1.Self-massage along meridians and acupoints should be done before sleep every night. It is especially effective in treating insomnia caused by mental stresses, environmental disturbances and sleep cycle changes as well as jetlag.

2.Care should be taken to keep a moderate diet, rest at regular times, alternate work with rest and in general keep good sleep habits.

3. Attempts should be made to do regular and appropriate physical work and physical exercise to strengthen overall health.

Section 9 Constipation

Introduction

Constipation is a symptom referring to the retention of dry feces in the intestine for over two days, usually marked by hard feces and difficulty in defecation. The causes of constipation are various. Constipation is caused mainly by the dryness of the feces caused by prolonged retention in the intestines and excessive absorption of fluid in the feces resulting from weakness in defecation, insufficient stimulation to the intestines, dysfunction of the nerves.

Traditional Chinese medicine holds that constipation is due mainly to a dysfunction of the stomach and intestines in transporting, which leads to retention of dry heat in the stomach and intestines that consumes body fluid and causes emotional upset, stagnant *qi* and abnormal changes in dredging and descending.

The Symptoms of Constipation

The usual symptoms are dry feces, difficulty in defecation, lack of defecation for over two days, accompanied by abdominal distension, belching, poor appetite, headache, vertigo, restless sleep, dysphoria, a susceptibility to rage and scanty yellow urine. Prolonged constipation may lead to hemorrhoids, anal cracks, as well as other problems.

Manipulations for Self-Massage Along Meridians and Acupoints

1. Pressing Zhongwan (CV 12) and Qihai Points (CV 6)
Performance: Supination with abdomen relaxed and knees and the hips bent. The index

and middle fingers of one hand press Zhongwan (located four *cun* above the navel) and Qihai (located 1.5 *cun* below the navel) repeatedly for about one minute respectively (see Fig. 1).

2. Pressing the Daheng Point (SP 15)

Performance: Supination. The index and middle fingers of both hands press Daheng (located four *cun* lateral to the navel and directly below the nipple, lateral to the abdominal rectus) simultaneously for about two minutes (see Fig. 2).

Among the three acupoints mentioned above, Zhongwan and Qihai are located on the conception vessel and Daheng on the spleen meridian. So this method is effective in dredging meridians and regulating the stomach and intestines.

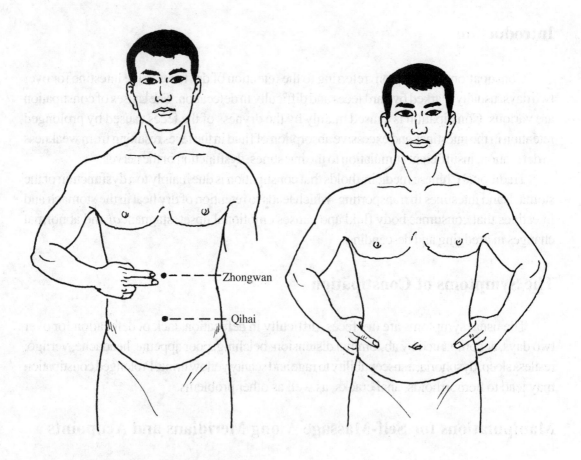

Zhongwan

Qihai

Fig. 1 Pressing Zhongwan and Qihai   **Fig. 2 Pressing Daheng**

3. Massaging the Abdomen

Performance: Supination with relaxed abdomen, and knees and hips bent. Breathing is natural. One hand is placed over the other to massage the abdomen, centering around the navel and the middle and lower part, massaging clockwise from the right to the left for about two minutes (see Fig. 3).

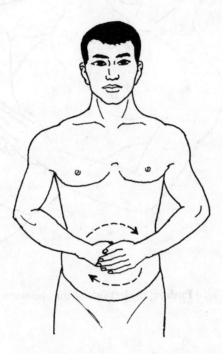

Fig. 3 Massaging the abdomen

4. Pushing the Left Side of the Abdomen

Performance: Supination with relaxed abdomen, knees bent and natural breathing. The left palm and fingers are placed on the upper part of the left side of the abdomen, and the right hand is placed on the back of the left hand. Then both hands together push and press for about two minutes (see Fig. 4).

Note: The pushing and pressing of the abdomen should be done gently and slowly. The manipulation is light and shallow at first and then heavy and deep until a comfortable sensation is felt.

These two methods are effective in promoting the peristalsis of the intestines and lubricating the intestines to ease defecation.

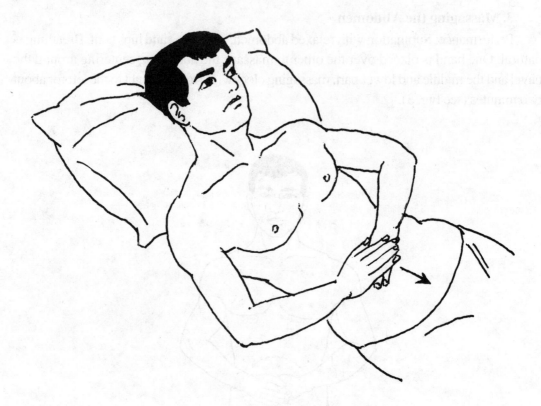

Fig. 4 Pushing the left side of the abdomen

5. Lifting the Anus

① Performance: Sitting position or supination. Both eyes are slightly closed with the tip of the tongue touching the upper palate, the mind calm and the body relaxed. Then the anus is slowly contracted, lifted and relaxed. This exercise is done repeatedly for about three minutes at a time.

② Effect: This technique can promote peristalsis of the intestines and defecation.

6. Stroking Baliao Acupoints

① Performance: Sitting position with the head and back leaning forward. The fingers of both hands are closed and placed over the posterior sacral foramens, the first of which is known as Shangliao (BL 31), the second Ciliao (BL 32), the third Zhongliao (BL 33) and the fourth Xialiao (BL 34). The stroking is done from the upper to the lower repeatedly for about three minutes (see Fig. 5).

② Effect: This method can calm the mind and eliminate dryness-heat.

7. Percussing the Abdomen

① Performance: Supination with a relaxed abdomen and natural stretching of the hips and knees. The fingers of both hands are relaxed to bend naturally. The tips of the fingers are used to percuss the abdomen lightly, especially the lower part of the left side, for about two minutes (see Fig. 6).

Note: The technique should be steady, flexible, light, swift and elastic.

② Effect: Dredges and smoothes the stomach and intestines.

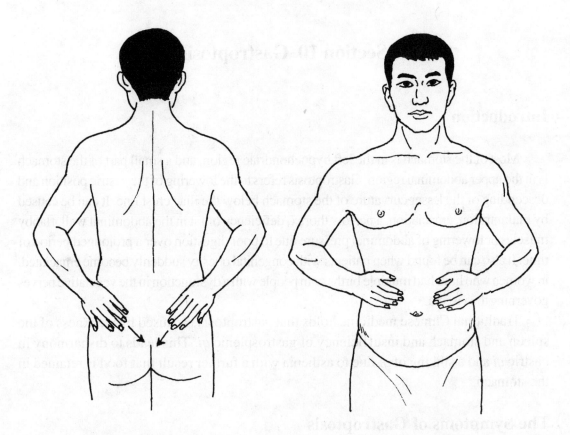

Fig. 5 Stroking Baliao   **Fig. 6 Percussing the abdomen**

Notes:

1. Self-massage along meridians and acupoints should be done once in the morning and once in the evening every day. It is effective in preventing and treating habitual constipation and functional constipation.

2. The patient should follow the habit of having a bowel movement every day even if there is no desire for defecation.

3. The diet should be moderate. The patient should eat more vegetables, fruits and food with more fibers.

4. Keep in a good mood and participate in appropriate physical work and exercise.

5. Do not do self-massage along meridians and acupoints on the abdomen for one and a half hours before or after a meal.

Section 10 Gastroptosis

Introduction

Most of the stomach is in the left hypochondriac region, and a small part of the stomach is in the upper abdominal region. Gastroptosis refers to the lowering of the gastric position and descending of the lesser curvature of the stomach below the iliac crest line. It can be caused by malnutrition, emaciation, a narrow thorax, deficiency of fat in the abdominal wall, flabby muscles or lowering of abdominal pressure due to poor digestion over a prolonged period of time. It also can be found when patients with congenital obesity suddenly become emaciated, in women who have had multiple births or in people with a dysfunction in the vegetative nerves governing the viscera.

Traditional Chinese medicine holds that gastroptosis is caused by weakness of the spleen and stomach and insufficiency of gastrosplenic *qi*. This leads to disharmony in gastric *qi* and a sinking of *qi* due to asthenia with a further result that food is retained in the stomach.

The Symptoms of Gastroptosis

At the early stage there are no symptoms. Patients with serious gastroptosis who have suffered the condition over a longer period of time may have the sensation of upper abdominal distension and sinking when standing up after meal. In most cases, these symptoms are alleviated when the patient lies flat. The usual symptoms of gastroptosis include emaciation, fatigue, poor appetite and colic, accompanied by belching, acid reflux or vomiting, sometimes also accompanied by palpitations, vertigo, insomnia, abitter taste in the mouth and dry throat as well as diarrhea.

Manipulations for Self-Massage Along Meridians and Acupoints

1. Pressing Jiuwei (CV 15), Zhongwan (CV 12), Qihai (CV 6) and Tianshu (ST 25) Points.

① Performance: Supination with hips and knees bent, relaxed abdomen and natural breathing. The index and middle fingers of one hand press Jiuwei (located in the depression below the sternum), Zhongwan (located four *cun* above the navel) and Qihai (located 1.5 *cun* below the navel) (see Fig. 1) for two minutes respectively (see Fig. 2).

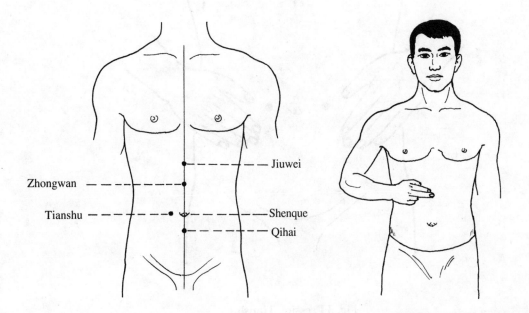

<table>
<tr><td>Fig. 1 Acupoints</td><td>Fig. 2 Pressing the acupoints illustrated in Fig. 1</td></tr>
</table>

Then the index and middle fingers of both hands simultaneously press Tianshu (located two *cun* lateral to the navel) for two minutes (see Fig. 3).

② Effect: Jiuwei, Zhongwan and Qihai are located on the conception vessel, and Tianshu is located on the stomach meridian. So this method is effective in strengthening the spleen and stomach and eliminating abdominal distension.

2. Pushing and Pressing the Abdomen

Performance: Supination with hips and knees bent and relaxed abdomen. The right palm is placed over the navel and the left palm is put on the back of the right hand. Both hands knead forcefully and clockwise from the right to the upper part and from the left to the lower part for three minutes. The kneading is light at first and then heavy until a warm and comfortable sensation is felt in the abdomen (see Fig. 4).

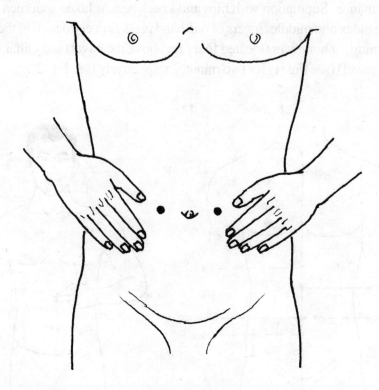

Fig. 3 Pressing Tianshu

3. Pushing and Holding the Fundus (lower end of the stomach)

Performance: Supination with knees bent and abdomen relaxed. The ulnar side of the right palm and fingers are placed at the lower border of the stomach on the left side with the aid of the left hand. Push the stomach in coordination with the breath. In exhalation, the pushing of the fundus (end opposite to the opening) of the stomach begins slowly from the pubic region on the left side of the lower abdomen to the navel; on inhalation, the abdomen and stomach are relaxed. The pushing is done repeatedly for about three minutes (see Fig. 5).

Note: The manipulation should be light at first and then heavy. The pushing is slow and deep. Care should be taken to avoid rapid and sudden pushing.

This method is effective in promoting digestion and lifting the stomach.

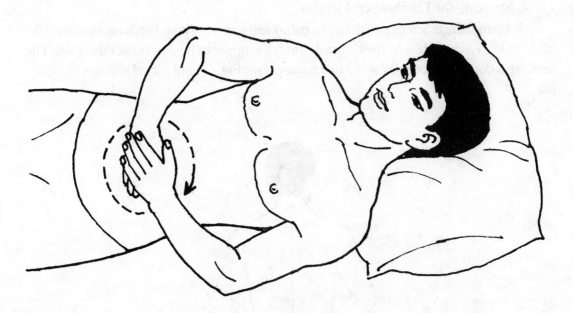

Fig. 4 Pushing and kneading the abdomen

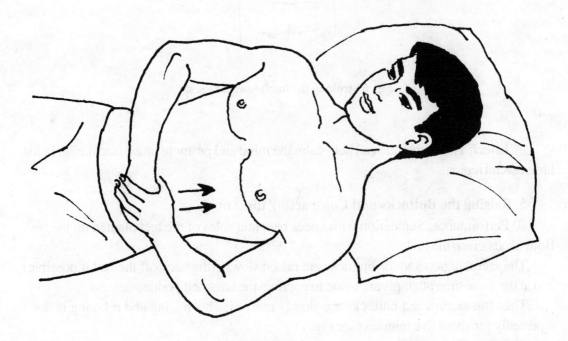

Fig. 5 Pushing and holding the lower end of the stomach

4. Stroking the Lumbosacral Region

① Performance: Sitting position. The palms and fingers of both hands are placed on the back, as high as possible, to stroke firmly from the upper to the lumbosacral region. The stroking is done repeatedly for about two minutes (see Fig. 6) until a local warm sensation is felt.

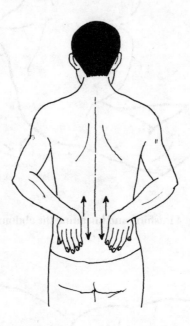

Fig. 6 Stroking the lumbosacral region

② Effect: This technique can help calm the mind and promote blood circulation in the lumbosacral region.

5. Raising the Buttocks and Contracting the Anus

① Performance: Supination with knees bent and soles of the feet planted on the bed. Both hands grasp the bed.

The sacral region and the buttocks are raised slowly (the back off the bed if possible) and at the same time attempts are made to contract the anus and perineum.

Then the sacrum and buttocks are slowly relaxed. This raising and relaxing is done repeatedly for about five minutes (see Fig. 7).

② Effect: This method can strengthen the abdominal muscles and improve the functions of the stomach and intestines.

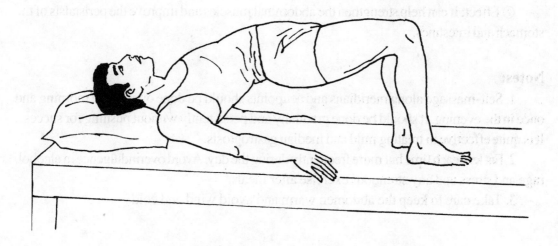

Fig. 7 Raising the buttocks and contracting the anus

6. Doing Sit-Ups

① Performance: Supination with legs straight. The head, chest and upper limbs move to the sit-up position on the inhalation and lie back down on the exhalation. Don't hold the breath but maintain regular breathing. Do sit-ups repeatedly for about two minutes (see Fig. 8).

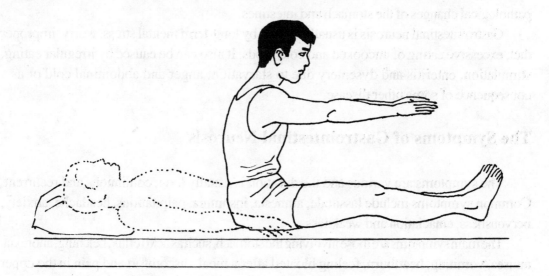

Fig. 8 Doing sit-ups

② Effect: It can help strengthen the abdominal muscles and improve the peristalsis of the stomach and intestines.

Notes:

1. Self-massage along meridians and acupoints should be done once in the morning and once in the evening. It should be done gradually and persistently without pushing for success. It is quite effective in treating mild and median gastroptosis.

2. Eat less each time but more frequently during the day. Avoid overindulgence in alcohol, rage and stress and any strenuous exercise after meals.

3. Take care to keep the abdomen warm and avoid wind and cold.

Section 11 Gastrointestinal Neurosis

Introduction

Gastrointestinal neurosis, usually seen among young and middle-aged women, refers to dysfunction of the stomach or intestines due to disturbance of the higher nerves without organic pathological changes of the stomach and intestines.

Gastrointestinal neurosis is usually caused by long-term mental stress, worry, improper diet, excessive eating of uncooked and cold foods. It also can be caused by irregular eating; stimulation, enteritis and dysentery due to starvation; anger and abdominal cold or as a consequence of some other disease.

The Symptoms of Gastrointestinal Neurosis

The symptoms are various and the duration is usually long, continuous and recurrent. Common symptoms include lassitude, amnesia, insomnia, palpitations, headache, anxiety, nervousness, emaciation and weakness.

The main symptoms are those involving the stomach, such as acid reflux, belching, anorexia, nausea, vomiting, heartburn, feeling bloated after a meal, discomfort and pain in the upper abdomen.

The symptoms involving the intestines include abdominal pain or discomfort, abdominal distension, gas, diarrhea and constipation.

Manipulations for Self-Massage Along Meridians and Acupoints

1. Pressing the Abdomen

① Performance: Supination with hips and knees bent and abdomen relaxed. The fingers of both hands are open and one hand is placed on the other on the abdomen. Centering on the navel, the hands press clockwise and counterclockwise on the middle and lower abdomen for two minutes respectively (see Fig. 1). Then the pressing extends to the whole body and is continued for one minute until a local warm and comfortable sensation is felt.

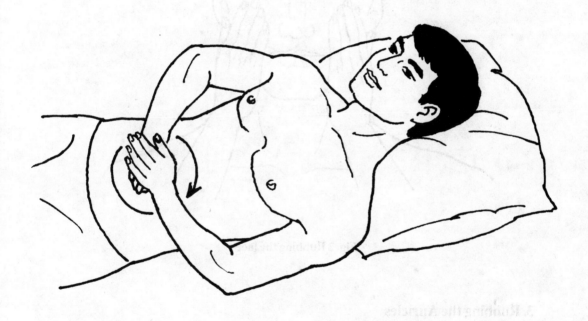

Fig. 1 Pressing the abdomen

② Effect: This technique may smooth intestinal and gastric *qi* activity, stop pain, ease distension and improve appetite.

2. Rubbing the Face

Performance: Sitting position with head and face relaxed. Moving counterclockwise, the palms and fingers rub their side of the face from the side of the nose to the eye and forehead like washing the face. This is done for two minutes (see Fig. 2).

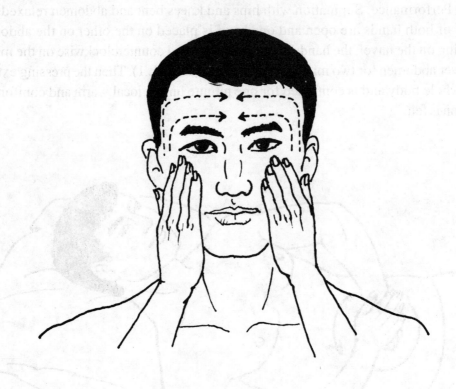

Fig. 2 Rubbing the face

3. Rubbing the Auricles

Performance: Sitting position. The thumbs and index fingers hold the auricles on the same side of the head and rub from the tip of the ear along the lateral and inferior side to the earlobe. Such rubbing is done for about two minutes (see Fig. 3) until a feverish sensation is felt in the skin of the earlobes, helix and auricles.

These two methods are effective in dredging the meridians, clearing the head and improving eyesight as well as calming the mind.

4. Pressing the Zusanli Point (ST 36)

Performance: Sitting position. The thumbs simultaneously or respectively press Zusanli [located three *cun* below Xiyan (ST 35) and about one transverse finger lateral to the tibia] on the same side of the leg until a local aching, numb and distending sensation is felt. The curative effect will be better if the sensation radiates to the toes (see Fig. 4).

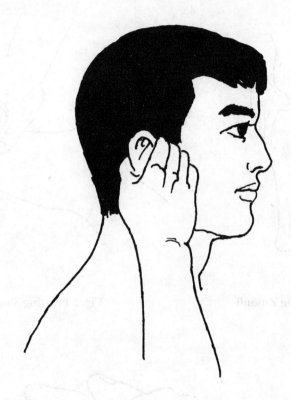

Fig. 3 Rubbing the auricle

5. Pressing the Taichong Point (LR 3)

Performance: Sitting position. The thumbs of both hands press Taichong (located 1.5 *cun* above the first and second interphalangeal space on the dorsum of the foot) for two minutes until a local aching, numb and distending sensation is felt (see Fig. 5).

6. Pressing the Neiguan Point (PC 6)

Performance: Sitting position. The thumb presses Neiguan (located two *cun* directly above the wrist transverse crease and between two tendons) on the opposite arm for one minute until a local aching, numb and distending sensation is felt (see Fig. 6).

Among these acupoints, Zusanli is located on the stomach meridian, Taichong on the liver meridian and Neiguan on the pericardium meridian. The pressing of these three acupoints is effective in helping the communications among meridians, dredging the intestines and stomach as well as easing distension and relieving pain.

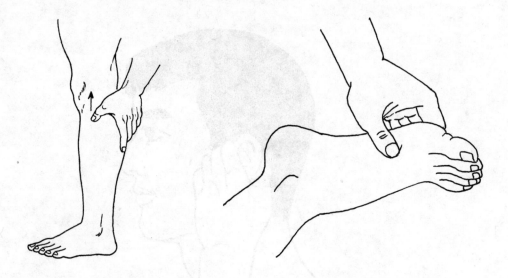

Fig. 4 Pressing Zusanli   **Fig. 5 Pressing Taichong**

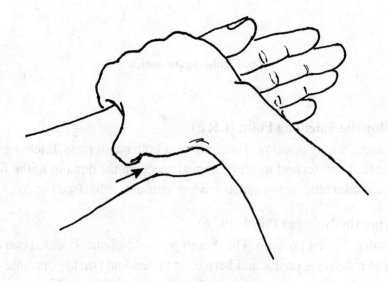

Fig. 6 Pressing Neiguan

7. Stroking the Lumbosacral Region

① Performance: Sitting position with a slight forward bending of the waist. The closed hands are put on the skin of the waist and back. Then stroke from the upper part to the lumbosacral region for about two minutes until the skin in the area turns reddish and warm sensation is felt (see Fig. 7).

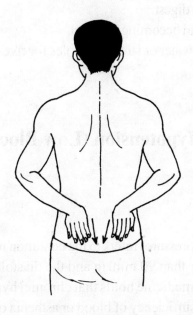

Fig. 7 Stroking the lumbosacral region

② Effect: This method can help warm and dredge meridians as well as regulate *qi* and blood.

8. Regulating Respiration

① Performance: Supination. Gentle abdominal breathing is performed. On the inhalation, the abdomen is contracted; while on the exhalation the abdomen expands. This method of respiration is practiced for about three minutes.

② Effect: This technique can smooth intestinal and gastric *qi* activity, relieve pain and ease distension.

Notes:

1. Self-massage along meridians and acupoints is done one or two times a day and

continued for 24 days. Then it may be done once every other day according to the pathological condition of the patient until all the symptoms have disappeared.

2. Massaging of the acupoints located on the abdomen should be gentle and slow, avoiding rough pressing. Do not do it one hour before or after a meal.

3. Care should be taken to keep a proper diet, a good mood and regular daily activities as well as to avoid smoking, drinking of alcohol and eating pungent, uncooked and cold foods or all foods that are difficult to digest.

4. Avoid catching cold and becoming stressed.

5. Soak the feet in warm water or stroke the soles for five to ten minutes before sleep.

Section 12 Hypotension (Low Blood Pressure)

Introduction

Hypotension (low blood pressure) refers to the condition in which the systolic pressure of the brachial artery is lower than 90 mmHg and the diastolic pressure is lower than 60 mmHg. Traditional Chinese medicine holds that chronici hypotension is usually caused by asthenia of *qi* and *yang*, insufficiency of blood or asthenia of both *qi* and *yin*.

The Symptoms of Hypotension

Acute hypotension is marked by sudden and obvious lowering of blood pressure, often accompanied by syncope and coma. So acute hypotension is not included in the indication of self-massage along meridians and acupoints.

Chronic hypotension usually shows no subjective symptoms. A few commonly seen symptoms are dizziness, distension of the head, vertigo, profuse sweating, palpitations, shortness of breath, a cold sensation in the arms and legs and general lassitude. Self-massage along meridians and acupoints is applicable for the treatment of chronic hypotension.

Manipulations for Self-Massage Along Meridians and Acupoints

1. Pressing the Suliao Point (GV 25)

① Performance: Sitting position. The middle finger of the right hand presses Suliao (located on the middle of the nose tip) for about one minute (see Fig. 1) until a local aching and distending sensation is felt (see Fig. 2).

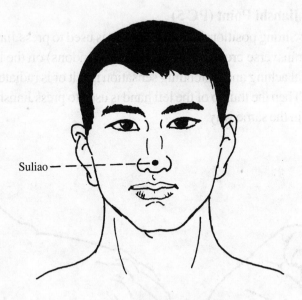

Fig. 1 Suliao

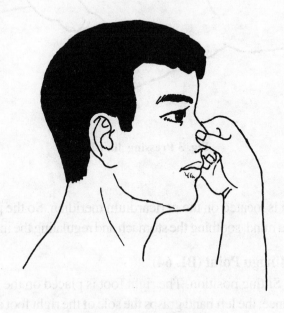

Fig. 2 Pressing Suliao

The manipulation should be gentle and moderate.

② Effect: Suliao is located on the governor vessel and is the key acupoint for the treatment of hypotension. So this method is effective in opening orifice and has general curative effect.

2. Pressing the Jianshi Point (PC 5)

① Performance: Sitting position. The right thumb is used to press Jianshi (located three *cun* above the wrist transverse crease and between two tendons) on the left hand for about one minute until a local aching and distending sensation is felt or is radiated to the upper arm and hand (see Fig. 3). Then the thumb of the left hand is used to press Jianshi on the right hand for about one minute in the same way.

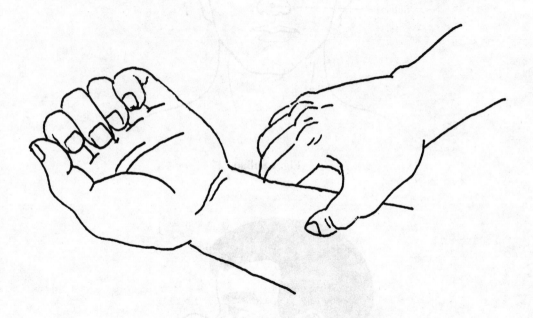

Fig. 3 Pressing Jianshi

② Effect: Jianshi is located on the pericardium meridian. So the pressing of Jianshi is effective in calming the mind, soothing the stomach and regulating the intestines.

3. Pressing the Jinggu Point (BL 64)

① Performance: Sitting position. The right foot is placed on the left leg and the right hand grasps the right knee; the left hand grasps the sole of the right foot and the middle finger is used to press Jinggu (located in the depression lateral to the fifth tuberosity of the metatarsal bone) (see Fig. 4) obliquely upward and vertically for about one minute (see Fig. 5). Then the middle finger of the right hand presses Jinggu on the left foot for about one minute.

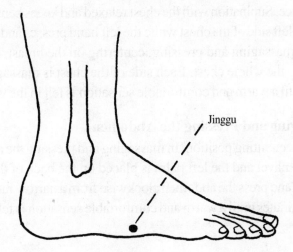

Fig. 4 Jinggu

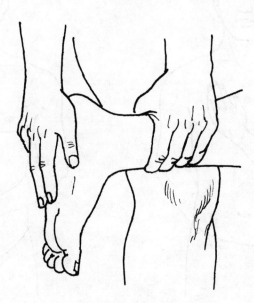

Fig. 5 Pressing Jinggu

② Effect: Jinggu is located on the bladder meridian. So pressing Jinggu is effective in calming the mind, clearing the head and improving eyesight.

4. Massaging and Pressing the Chest

Performance: Supination with the chest relaxed and knees bent. The right hand massages and presses the left side of the chest while the left hand presses and massages the right side of the chest. The massaging and pressing, centering on the breast, is done clockwise from a narrow range to the whole chest. Each side of the chest is massaged and pressed for about two minutes until a warm and comfortable sensation is felt in the whole chest (see Fig. 6).

5. Massaging and Pressing the Abdomen

Performance: Sitting position. In massaging and pressing the abdomen, the right palm is placed over the navel and the left palm is placed on the back of the right hand. Both hands firmly massage and press the abdomen clockwise from a narrow range to the whole abdomen for about two minutes until a warm and comfortable sensation is felt in the abdomen (see Fig. 7).

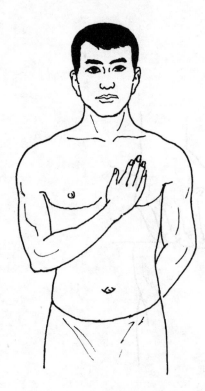
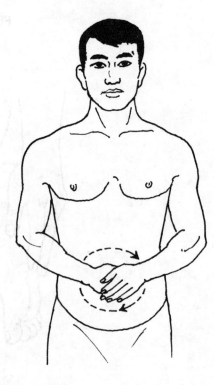

Fig. 6 Massaging and pressing the chest   **Fig. 7 Massaging and pressing the abdomen**

The methods mentioned above are effective in dredging the meridians, strengthening the tension of the blood vessels, promoting blood circulation and lifting blood pressure.

6. Rubbing the Auricles

① Performance: Sitting position. The thumbs and index fingers of both hands hold the outside of the ears on each side respectively and rub the ears from their tips gradually to the earlobe for about two minutes (see Fig. 8). The rubbing of the ears is continued till warm sensation is felt in the skin of the earlobes, helix and auricles.

② Effect: This technique can smooth tendons, activate collaterals, clear the head and improve eyesight. Apart from refreshing the brain, this method is also effective in dispersing stagnant liver *qi*, soothing the gallbladder, increasing blood pressure and strengthening immunity.

7. Stroking the Baliao Point

① Performance: Sitting position with a forward leaning of the head. The palms and fingers of both hands are placed on Baliao (located in the first, second, third and fourth posterior sacral foramens) on each side (see Fig. 9). The stroking is done from the upper region to the lower region for about three minutes (see Fig. 10).

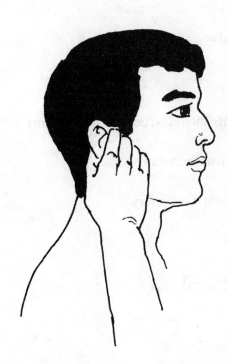

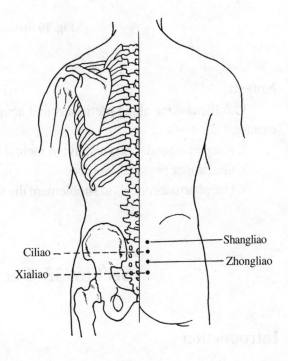

Ciliao
Xialiao
Shangliao
Zhongliao

Fig. 8 Rubbing the auricles   **Fig. 9 Baliao (posterior sacral foramens)**

② Effect: Baliao acupoints are located on the bladder meridian. So the stimulation of these acupoints is effective in regulating meridians and activating blood as well as strengthening the waist and supplementing kidney.

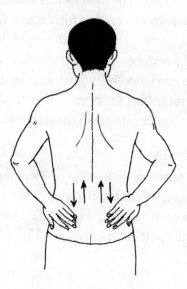

Fig. 10 Stroking Baliao

Notes:

1. Self-massage along meridians and acuppoints should be done in the morning and evening.

2. Keep in a good mood and avoid mental aggravation and stress.

3. Get proper physical exercise.

4. Use pharmaceuticals to supplement the treatment if necessary.

Section 13 Facial Paralysis

Introduction

The facial paralysis included in this section is peripheral facial paralysis due to acute nonsuppurating inflammation of the facial nerves in the stylomastoid foramen. It is generally believed that it is caused by ischemic edema of the nerves due to spasms of the local nutrient vessels caused by wind and cold. It may also be caused by local viral infections. Also, chronic tympanitis and mastoiditis can lead to secondary facial paralysis.

Traditional Chinese medicine holds that facial paralysis is caused by stagnation of the meridians, malnutrition of the tendons and vessels due to cold and wind attacking the face when *qi* and blood are insufficient.

The Symptoms of Facial Paralysis

Usually patients find that the face is distorted to one side, the eyes cannot close and the mouth hangs awry when they get up or wash or gargle in the morning. In a few cases a patient feels discomfort in the affected part before the onset of facial paralysis. The usual symptoms are a painful sensation below the ear or over the mastoid region on the affected side, onset of a blank facial expression, inability to close the eyes, tearing problems, inability to frown, distortion of the corner of the mouth toward the healthy side, a shallowness in the nasolabial groove, leakage of air from the mouth when speaking and difficulty in bulging the mouth as well as a reduction in the ability to taste or a loss of that ability in the front two-thirds of the tongue on the affected side as well as a painful intolerance for sound.

Self-Massage Along Meridians and Acupoints

1. Pushing and Massaging the Face
Performance: Sitting position with the face relaxed. The palms and the fingers of both hands rub together until they are warm. Then the palms and the fingers are used to rub the face from the lower jaw to the area around the mouth, the nose, the orbit and the forehead, especially the affected part. The rubbing is done repeatedly for about three minutes (see Fig. 1).

2. Pushing and Massaging the Affected Rregion
Performance: Sitting position. The thumb of one hand is placed on the corner of the mouth on the affected side to push forcefully toward the earlobe. Such a manipulation is continued for about two minutes (see Fig. 2).

These two methods are effective in promoting facial blood circulation.

3. Pressing the Taiyang Point (EX-HN 5)
Performance: Sitting position. The thumb of one hand is used to press Taiyang (located

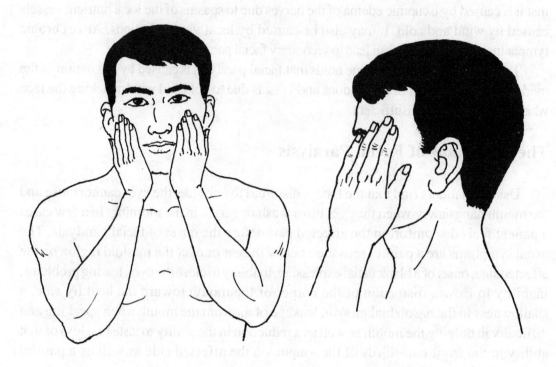

Fig. 1 Pushing and massaging the face   **Fig. 2 Pushing and massaging the affected part**

in the depression one *cun* lateral between the end of the eyebrow and the outer canthus) for about a minute (see Fig. 3).

4. Pressing the Jiache Point (ST 6)

Performance: Sitting position. The middle finger of one hand is used to press Jiache (located one transverse finger above the mandibular angle and at the prominence of masseter when one grits the teeth) on the affected side for about a minute (see Fig. 4).

5. Pressing the Fengchi Point (GB 20)

Performance: Sitting position. The thumbs of both hands are each placed at Fengchi (located below the occipital bone, parallel to the lower border of the sternocleidomastoid muscle and in the depression lateral to the prominence of the neck) (see Fig. 5) to press for about a minute (see Fig. 6).

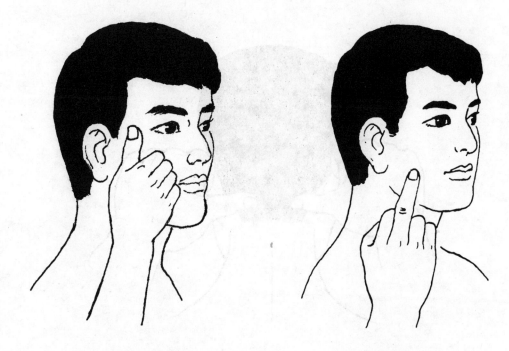

Fig. 3 Pressing Taiyang   **Fig. 4 Pressing Jiache**

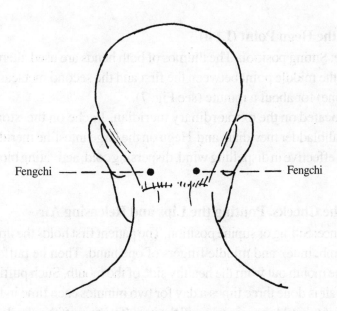

Fengchi   Fengchi

Fig. 5 Fengchi

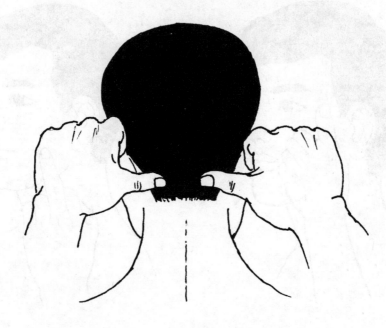

Fig. 6 Pressing Fengchi

6. Pressing the Hegu Point (LI 4)

Performance: Sitting position. The thumbs of both hands are used alternatively to press Hegu (located in the middle point between the first and the second metacarpus and slightly near the second one) for about a minute (see Fig. 7).

Taiyang is located on the extraordinary meridian, Jiache on the stomach meridian, Fengchi on the gallbladder meridian, and Hegu on the large intestine meridian. So pressing these acupoints is effective in dispelling wind, dispersing cold, activating blood and dredging meridians.

7. Puffing the Cheeks, Pouting the Lips and Releasing Air

① Performance: Sitting or supine position. The patient first holds the lips on the affected side with the thumb, index and middle fingers of one hand. Then he puffs the cheeks and blows the air in the mouth out from the healthy side of the mouth. Such puffing of the cheeks and releasing the air is done three times a day for two minutes each time in front of a mirror. Every day the patient should consciously pull the nose, frown, puff the cheeks, pout the mouth and roll the tongue around inside the cheeks. Such practice should be done for two minutes each time (see Fig. 8).

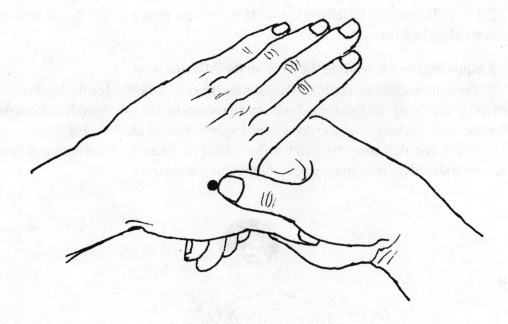

Fig. 7 Pressing Hegu

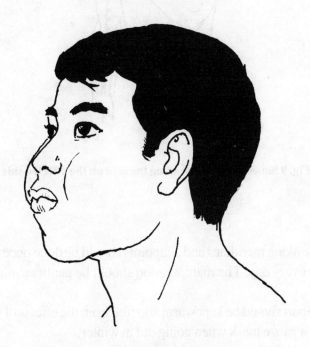

Fig. 8 Puffing cheeks, pouting the lips and releasing air

② Effect: This method is effective to smooth the tendons, dredge collaterals and promote movement of the facial muscles.

8. Squeezing and Kneading the Arm on the Affected Side

① Performance: Sitting position. The palm and fingers of the hand on the healthy side pinch and knead the arm on the affected side from the shoulder along the lateral border of the limb to the wrist. Such massage should be done for about two minutes (see Fig. 9).

② Effect: The triple energizer meridian flows along the lateral border of the upper limb. So this method is effective in promoting the flow of triple energizer *qi*.

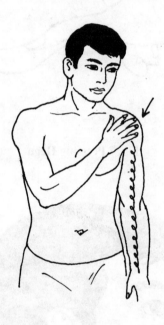

Fig. 9 Squeezing and kneading the arm on the affected side

Notes:

1. Self-massage along meridians and acupoints should be done once in the morning and once in the evening every day. The manipulation should be gentle, avoiding damage to the facial skin.

2. The affected part should be kept warm and free from the effects of wind and cold. The patient should wear a gauze mask when going out in winter.

3. Care should be taken to prevent infection of the cornea on the affected side by using eye drops and ointments.

Section 14 Temporomandibular Joint Syndrome

Introduction

Temporomandibular joint syndrome is a dysfunctional disease caused by disorders in the joints, muscles and nerves. The temporomandibular joint (the joints on either side of the face connecting the lower jaw with the skull) is the only mobile joint in the facial region.

Temporomandibular joint syndrome is caused by malposition or malformation of the teeth, excessively worn teeth, long-term chewing on one side, traumatic injury of the temporomandibular joint, violent yawning and chewing or the effects of cold and wind. These can lead to the impairment of the temporomandibular joint through damage to muscles, tendons and nerves.

The onset is usually slow. It is seen often among middle-aged and young women, frequently involving one side, occasionally involving both sides.

The Symptoms of Temporomandibular Joint Syndrome

The usual symptoms are restrictions in opening the mouth and pain in the joints when opening the mouth or chewing, sometimes accompanied by a snapping feeling. In severe cases there may appear weakness of the masseter (muscle raising the lower jaw) and obvious tenderness anterior to the tragus (prominence in front of opening of the ear). In a few cases there are the symptoms of dysacusis (loss of the ability to interpret sounds) as well as headache and vertigo due to pressure on the temporal nerve and tympanic cord nerve next to the condyloid process.

Self-Massage Along Meridians and Acupoints

1. Pushing and Kneading the Xiaguan Point (ST 7)
Performance: Sitting position. The index and middle fingers of one hand push and knead Xiaguan (located in the depression between the zygomatic arch and the mandibular notch) at the affected side for about a minute (see Fig. 1).

2. Pushing and Kneading the Jiache Point (ST 6)
Performance: Sitting position. The index and middle fingers of one hand push and knead

Jiache (located one transverse finger above the mandibular angle or at the prominence of the masseter) for about a minute (see Fig. 2).

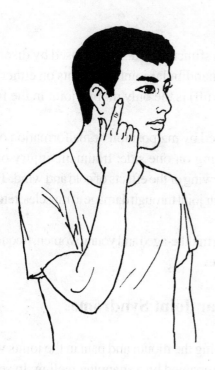

Fig. 1 Pushing and kneading Xiaguan

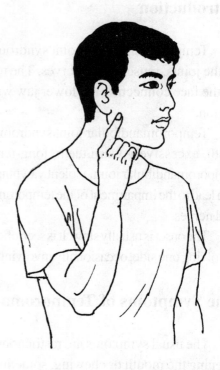

Fig. 2 Pushing and kneading Jiache

3. Pushing and Kneading the Yifeng Point (TE 17)

Performance: Sitting position. The thumb, index and middle fingers of one hand push and knead Yifeng (located behind the earlobe and in the depression between the mandibular angle and mastoid process) for about a minute (see Fig. 3).

Notes:

① The acupoints mentioned above should be simultaneously pushed and kneaded gently and slowly until a slight distending is felt in the acupoints and the temporal muscle and the muscles responsible for closing and opening the mouth are relaxed.

② In the pushing and kneading acupoints, efforts should be made to open and close the mouth slowly, evenly and according to the condition.

Among the acupoints mentioned above, Xiaguan and Jiache are located on the stomach meridian, and Yifeng on the triple energizer meridian. So the pushing and kneading of these acupoints are effective in relaxing the tendons, activating collaterals, relieving spasm and stopping pain.

4. Rubbing the Face

Performance: Sitting position. The palms and fingers are used to rub the face on either side from the mandibular angle to the ear and forehead as in washing the face for about two minutes (see Fig. 4).

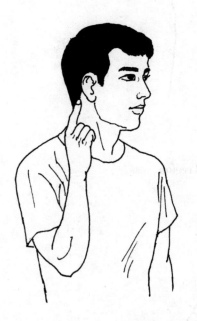

Fig. 3 Pushing and kneading Yifeng　　　　　　　**Fig. 4 Rubbing the face**

5. Kneading the Temporal Region

Performance: Sitting position. One hand holds the healthy side of the face and the heel of the palm of the other hand is used to knead the temporal region on the affected side for about two minutes until a warm sensation is felt in the affected part (see Fig. 5).

6. Percussing the Temporal Region

Performance: The fingers of both hands are slightly bent and the tips of the fingers are used to tap the temporal regions, like a bird pecking food, for about a minute (see Fig. 6). The percussion should be done swiftly and gently.

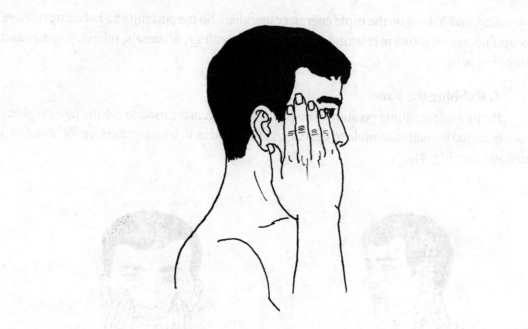

Fig. 5 Kneading the temporal region

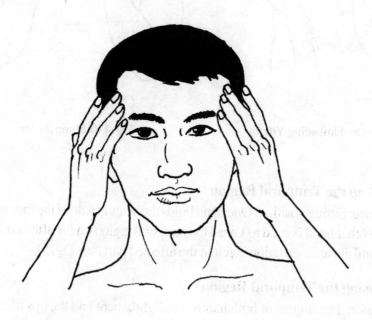

Fig. 6 Percussing the temporal region

These three methods are effective in stopping pain, easing inflammation and lubricating joints.

Notes:

1. According to clinical observations, temporomandibular joint syndrome is usually caused by spasms in the lateral pterygoid muscle, or by spasms in the lateral pterygoid muscle and masseter due to a relative displacement of the condyloid process in the articular disc. So the treatment should focus on relief of spasm and pain. Self-massage along meridians and acupoints is done once a day. It is effective in relieving spasms, stopping pain and easing inflammation. It is especially effective in the patient where the disease has been present a short time and symptoms are light.

2. Heat can be applied to the affect part with a warm towel or warm wax bag.

3. Avoid foods that are difficult to chew.

4. Correct bad chewing habits, such as long-term chewing on one side.

5. Self-massage along meridians and acupoints is not as effective if there is a fundamental problem with bone structure.

Section 15 Stiff Neck

Introduction

Stiff neck is a commonly encountered disease marked by spasms of the sternocleidomastoid muscle, trapezius muscle and levator muscle of the scapula as well as stiffness and restriction of the neck.

Stiff neck is usually caused by improper posture in sleep (such as when the head slips off the pillow or the pillow is too high or too low) which leads to long-term fatigue in the cervical muscles and stagnation in blood circulation which can result in reflex spasms of the cervical muscles on one side as well as a deviation in the neck. In some cases stiff neck is caused by an attack of cold and wind or trauma during sleep which leads to obstruction of the local meridians, stagnancy of *qi* and blood, malnutrition of local muscles and spasms in tendons and blood vessels.

The Symptoms of Stiff Neck

Usually the patient feels aching pain and stiffness on one side of the neck as well as difficulty in moving and rotating the head when he or she gets up in the morning. If the patient tries to move the head to a normal position, the pain becomes aggravated and can even involve the shoulder and back. Examination: Spasms of the muscles on one side of the neck, obvious tenderness, a palpable rope-like mass of tissue or nodule in the neck, restricted movement of the neck and tenderness at the inner angle of the scapula.

Self-Massage Along Meridians and Acupoints

1. Pressing and kneading the Fengchi point (GB 20)

Performance: Sitting position. The tips of the thumbs of both hands are used alternatively to press and knead Fengchi (located in the depression below the occipital tuberosity) for about one minute (see Fig. 1). The massage is light at first and then heavy.

Then the kneading technique is used to knead clockwise until a local aching, distending and comfortable sensation is felt. During the course of kneading, the head is rotated slowly several times.

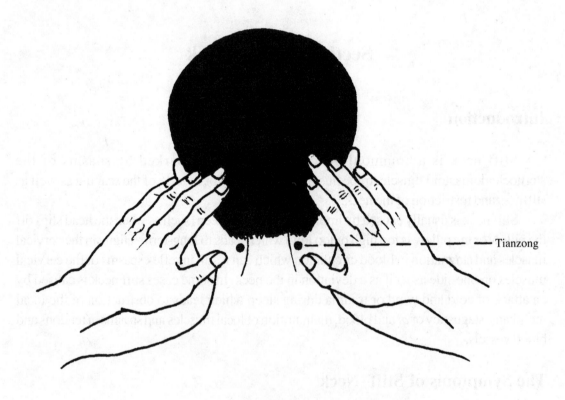

Tianzong

Fig. 1 Pressing and kneading Fengchi

2. Pressing and kneading the Jianjing point (GB 21)

Performance: Sitting position. The middle finger of one hand presses and kneads Jianjing (located on the middle point of the line connecting the seventh cervical vertebral process and the acromion and at the prominence of the shoulder) for about two minutes until a local aching and distending sensation is felt (see Fig. 2). Then the other side is pressed and kneaded in the same way.

3. Pressing and kneading Tianzong (SI 11)

Performance: Sitting position with the relaxation of the cervical muscles. One hand is placed on the shoulder of the other side, and the middle finger is used to press Tianzong (located in the middle of infraspinous fossa of the scapula) for two minutes until an aching and

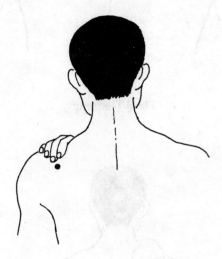

Fig. 2 Pressing and kneading Jianjing

distending sensation is felt in the shoulder and back and a limp or relaxed feeling is felt in the arm on the affected side (see Fig. 4).

When being kneaded and pressed, the neck should be rotated slowly starting in a small circle to a wider range until the neck feels less stiff, pain is alleivated and the movement of the head is improved.

Among the three acupoints mentioned above, Fengchi and Jianjing are located on the gallbladder meridian, and Tianzong on the small intestine meridian. Frequent pressing and kneading of these acupoints is effective in activating blood, dredging meridians, dispelling wind and relieving superficial pathogenic factors.

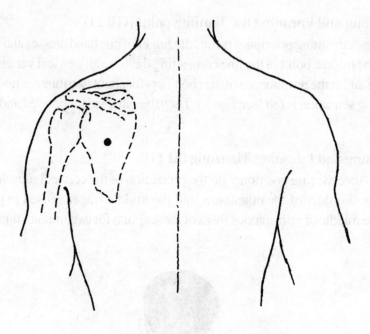

Fig. 3 Tianzong

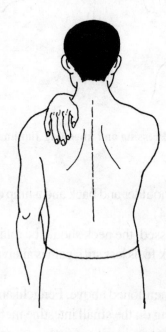

Fig. 4 Pressing and kneading Tianzong

4. Rubbing and Massaging the Neck

① Performance: Sitting position. The hand on the healthy side is raised up with palm open and four fingers close together. The palm is put on the back and sides of the cervical vertebrae to rub and massage for two minutes with the palm in close contact with the skin. The manipulation should be harmonious and rhythmic. The strength used for rubbing and massaging should be even and deep until a comfortable and warm sensation is felt (see Fig. 5). Then the other hand is used to rub and massage the neck the same way.

② Effect: This method can warm and dredge *qi* and blood, and relieve spasms and pain.

5. Kneading the Neck and Shoulder

① Performance: Sitting position. The palm of one hand is placed on the opposite side of the neck with fingers slightly bent. The index, middle, ring and little fingers with the heel of the

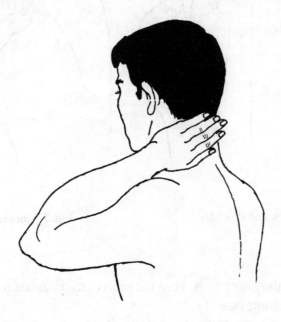

Fig. 5 Rubbing and massaging the neck

palm rhythmically knead from the neck to the acromion (outer end of the scapula to which the collarbone is attached) for about a minute. The kneading is light at first and then heavier, monitored to the tolerance of the patient until a comfortable sensation is felt (see Fig. 6). Then the other hand is used to knead the other side in the same way.

② Effect: This method dredge meridians and relieve spasm.

6. Patting the Neck

(1) Performance: Sitting position with neck and head relaxed.

① Squeezing and lifting the nape: The fingers of both hands intertwine to hold the nape

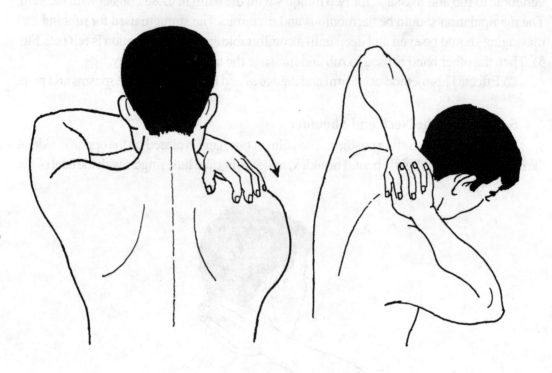

Fig. 6 Kneading the neck and shoulder   **Fig. 7 Squeezing and lifting the nape**

and the head leans slightly backward. Then the heels of the palm are used to squeeze and lift the nape for about a minute (see Fig. 7).

② Light patting of the neck: The hand on one side is raised over the chest with the slight bending of the five fingers to pat the other side of the neck from top to bottom for about one to two minutes (see Fig. 8). Then the other hand is used to pat the other side of the neck in the same way.

③ Moving the neck: When the cervical muscles are relaxed, the head and neck are bent forward, backward and to both sides. But such movement should be done slowly and gently, avoiding any sudden movement (see Fig. 9).

(2) Effect: This technique can help relax the tendon, activate blood, warm meridians and dredge collaterals.

Notes:

1. Self-massage along meridians and acupoints is done one or two times a day. Frequent massaging of the neck is effective in preventing and treating stiff neck.

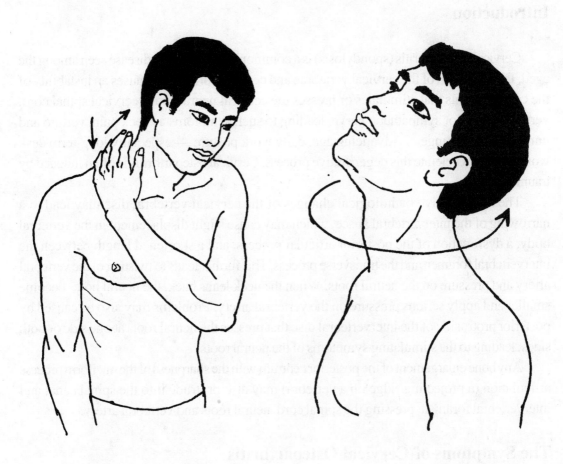

Fig. 8 Patting the neck   **Fig. 9 Moving the neck**

2. Stiff neck is a kind of acute injury of the soft tissues. Proper and timely treatment will ensure quick recovery without subsequent problems. However, recurrent relapses may lead to disease of the cervical vertebrae. So a stiff neck must be treated in time. If the curative effect is not remarkable, the patient should be examined at a hospital to see if other diseases may be involved.

3. Keep a proper sleeping position and find an appropriate pillow. A pillow should not be too high. Care, too, should be taken to keep the neck warm.

Section 16 Cervical Osteoarthritis

Introduction

Cervical osteoarthritis (spondylosis) is a commonly encountered disease seen among the aged. Degeneration of the cervical vertebrae and cervical soft tissues causes an instability of the cervical joints that stimulates or presses the cervical neural roots, cervical spinal cord, vertebral artery or sympathetic nerve, leading to such symptoms as neck pain, vertigo and numbness in the fingers. Advancing age, daily work posture — especially long-term desk work — may accelerate this degenerative process. Cervical osteoarthritis is often induced by traumatic injury.

The degenerative pathological changes of the cervical vertebral disc may lead to a narrowing of the intervertebral space, which may cause slight displacement in the vertebral body, a dysfunction of the posterior articular process, and a shortened length between the intervertebral foramen and the transverse process. This further leads to twisting of the vertebral artery and pressure on the neural roots. When the neck leans back, the neural holes become smaller and apply serious pressure on the vertebral artery. Problems may also be caused by posterior protrusion of the intervertebral disc that presses the neural roots at one side or both sides, leading to the stimulating symptoms of the neural roots.

Any bone enlargement of the posterior centrum with the sharpness of the unciform process articulation (a projecting ridge on a vertebra) may also protrude into the spinal canal and intervertebral foramen, pressing the spinal cord, neural roots and vertebral artery.

The Symptoms of Cervical Osteoarthritis

Cervical osteoarthritis is marked by slow onset except in the case of acute traumatic injury. At the primary stage, there is intermittent or continuous pain or discomfort in the neck. With the development of the pathological process, the symptoms are aggravated with radiating pain and numbness in the shoulder, neck, back, chest and upper limbs. The pain is worsened when sleeping, coughing, sneezing, defecating, working with the head bent or moving the neck. Clinically cervical osteoarthritis is divided into the following types:

1. Neural root type: The neural roots are pressed, leading to radiating pain on one side or both sides of the upper arms and numbness of the fingers.

2. Vertebral artery type: The cervical vertebral artery is twisted due to pressure and temporarily reduces or stagnates blood flow, consequently leading to an insufficient blood supply to the brain and resulting in headache, vertigo and even postural coma, etc.

3. Sympathetic nerve type: The sympathetic nerve is stimulated, leading to such symptoms as weakness of the eyelids, tearing problems, flushed cheeks, susceptibility to sweating, restlessness, fatigue and rapid heartbeat.

4. Spinal cord type: The spinal nerves are pressed, leading to numbness of the legs, unstable gait, pain in one side or both sides of the upper arms, numbness of the fingers, or even incontinence or paralysis in severe cases. Delayed treatment may result in a disability.

So cervical osteoarthritis is marked by slighter symptoms in the neck and more serious symptoms in other parts of the body; frequent involvement of the four limbs, head, trunk and even the whole body; and a poor prognosis in the spinal cord type with incontinence as well as paralysis.

Self-Massage Along Meridians and Acupoints

1. Squeezing and Kneading the Neck, Shoulders and Arms

① Performance: Sitting position. The thumb, index, middle, ring and little fingers of one hand pinch and knead along the bilateral sides of the cervical vertebral process and muscles in the affected upper limb. The squeezing and kneading are done repeatedly from the occipital region to the uppermost part of the back and muscles in both sides of the neck as well as the upper arm and forearm. In the region affected by pain, sometimes a palpable rope-like mass can be found. This is usually the focus of the disease and is also the main place to be squeezed and kneaded. The squeezing and kneading are done repeatedly for about five minutes (see Figs. 1 and 2). Then the other hand is used in the same way.

② Effect: This method can relax muscles, relieve spasm and stop pain.

2. Pressing and Kneading the Jianjing Point (GB 21)

Performance: Sitting position. The middle finger of one hand is used to press Jianjing (located on the middle point on the line connecting the seventh cervical vertebral spinous process with the acromion at the prominence of the shoulder) for about two minutes until a local aching and distending sensation is felt (see Fig. 3).

3. Pressing and Kneading the Fengchi Point (GB 20)

Performance: Sitting position. The thumbs of both hands are placed at Fengchi (located in the depression below the occipital tuberosity). They press gently at first and then more heavily for about two minutes (see Fig. 4).

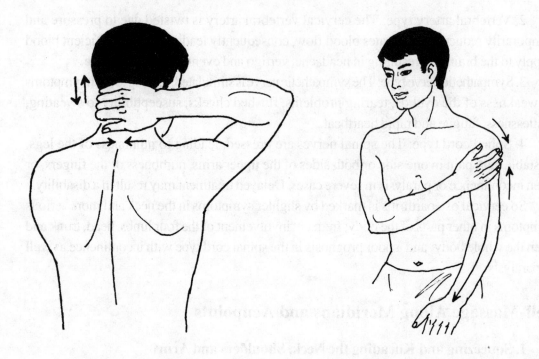

Fig. 1 Squeezing and kneading nape   **Fig. 2 Squeezing and kneading the shoulder and arm**

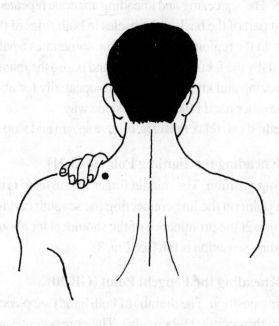

Fig. 3 Pressing and kneading Jianjing

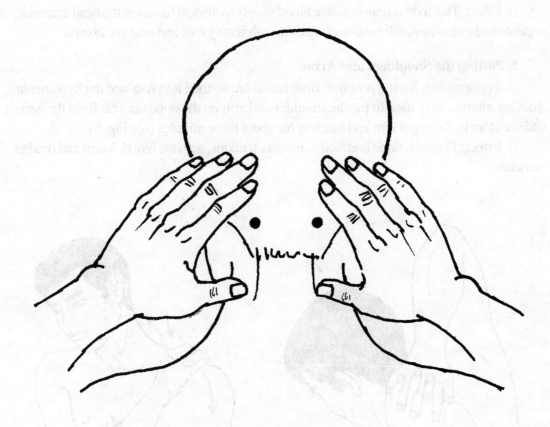

Fig. 4 Pressing and kneading Fengchi

Jianjing and Fengchi are located on the gallbladder meridian. So pressing Jianjing and Fengchi is effective in activating blood, dredging meridians, dispelling wind and relieving superficial pathogenic factors.

4. Squeezing and Lifting the Nape

① Performance: Sitting position. The fingers of both hands are intertwined to embrace the nape with a slight leaning back of the head. The heels of the palms and the fingers are used to squeeze and lift the muscles on both sides of the cervical spinous process. The squeezing and lifting massage is done gently at first and then forcibly and repeatedly from the top to the bottom part of the neck at a slow pace. At the same time the neck is bent forward and back and turned to the left and right 12 times (see Fig. 5).

The movement in the neck in each direction should be big but slow.

② Effect: This method can improve blood supply to the soft tissues in the head and neck, regulate body functions, relieve muscle spasms, lubricate joints and ease symptoms.

5. Patting the Shoulders and Arms

① Performance: Sitting position. Both hands are formed into fists and the hypothenar sides are alternatively used to pat the shoulder and arm on the opposite side from the nape and shoulder to the upper arm and forearm for about three minutes (see Fig. 6).

② Effect: This technique is effective to relax tendons, activate blood, warm and dredge meridians.

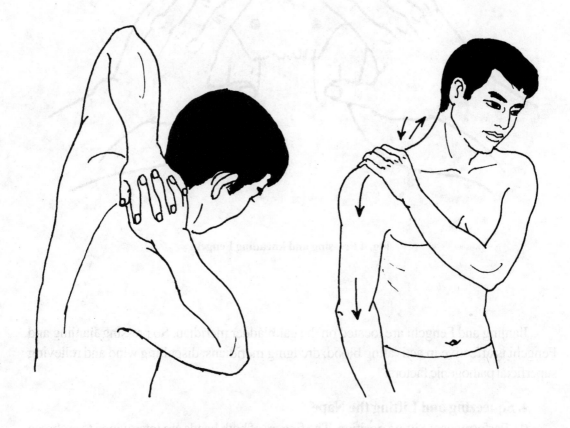

Fig. 5 Squeezing and lifting nape   Fig. 6 Patting the shoulders and arms

6. Rounding the Neck

① Performance: Sitting position. To relax the muscles in the neck, the neck is slowly rounded clockwise and counterclockwise for about three minutes (see Fig. 7).

② Effect: This method can help relax muscles and lubricate joints.

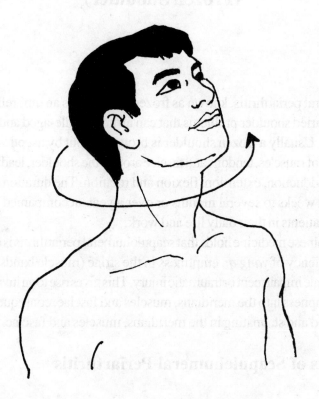

Fig. 7 Rounding the neck

Notes:

1. Self-massage along meridians and acupoints here should be done once in the morning and once in the evening every day following the methods mentioned above. It is effective in relaxing the muscles in the shoulder, promoting blood circulation, relaxing the tendons to activate blood, soothing the tendons to restore normal functions and relieving symptoms. It is especially effective in treating neural root type which involves 60 percent of the cervical osteoarthritis cases.

2. Care should be taken to avoid a long-term bending over of the head or neck into a fixed position. Pillows should be the right height. According to the physiological characteristics of the cervical vertebrae, the pillow should be as high as the height of a fist when one sleeps in a supine position and of a fist and a half when one sleeps on one's side.

3. Care should be taken to keep the neck and back warm and prevent wind and cold.

Section 17　Scapulohumeral Periarthritis
(Frozen Shoulder)

Introduction

Scapulohumeral periarthritis, known as frozen shoulder, is an umbrella term to describe the common and varied shoulder problems that can afflict middle-aged and older people. The causes are various. Usually a frozen shoulder is brought about by aseptic inflammation and extensive adhesion of muscles, tendons and fasciae around the shoulder, leading to confinement of the shoulder in adduction, extension, flexion and rotation. The duration of this disease can range from several weeks to several months or over a year, accompanied by much pain and inconvenience to patients in their daily life and work.

Traditional Chinese medicine holds that scapulohumeral periarthritis is caused by physical weakness, insufficiency of *yang qi*, emptiness in the striae (muscle bands), looseness of the defensive *qi* or chronic impairment or traumatic injury. This gives rise to an invasion of pathogenic wind, cold and dampness into the meridians, muscles and fasciae, consequently inhibiting the flow of *qi* and blood and stagnating in the meridians, muscles and fasciae.

The Symptoms of Scapulohumeral Periarthritis

This disease can be acute, but usually it is chronic and begins to be seen among people around the age of 50. At the primary stage the shoulder feels uncomfortable with non-localized pain that becomes worsened with movement. Gradually the shoulder feels stiff, and the pain becomes aggravated at night. Usually it is not related to changes in weather. Examination finds no swelling in the shoulder, no reddish change of the skin and no fever. Mild atrophy is found in some cases. The pain of this disease can cover a wide area, and tenderness is not confined to one spot. Clinically, tenderness can be found at the supraspinous muscle, infraspinous muscle, supraspinatus tendon (rotator cuff) connected with the greater tuberosity of the humerus as well as the region where the subdeltoid bursa and the biceps in the arm pass by the humeral tuberosity. "When the shoulder moves, its range is limited when the arm is raised, rotated inward, rotated outward or lifted away from the body.

Self-Massage Along Meridians and Acupoints

1. Pressing and Kneading the Shoulder

Performance: Sitting position. The opposite hand is put on the shoulder of the affected side with the thumb and palm heel on the front and the four fingers toward the back to repeatedly press and knead the muscles around the shoulder for about five minutes until a warm sensation is felt on the skin (see Fig. 1).

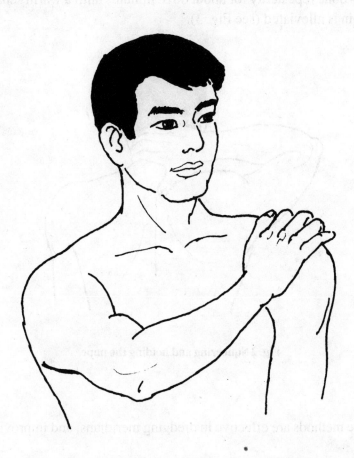

Fig. 1 Pressing and kneading the shoulder

2. Squeezing and Holding the Neck

Performance: Sitting position. The head leans slightly toward the healthy side, and the hand of the healthy side is put on the neck and back of the affected side. The palm and fingers are used to squeeze and hold for about three minutes until a warm sensation is felt on the skin (see Fig. 2).

3. Squeezing and Kneading Tenderness of the Shoulder and Arm

Performance: Sitting position. The opposite hand is placed on the upper arm of the affected side with the thumb in front and the four fingers in back. The thumb is used to pinch and knead the tenderness at the front part of the shoulder and the upper region of the arm, i.e., the long head or short head of the biceps muscle tendon of the arm. The squeezing and kneading is done repeatedly for about three minutes until a warm sensation is felt in the area and pain is alleviated (see Fig. 3).

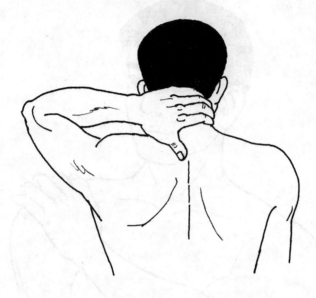

Fig. 2 Squeezing and holding the nape

These three methods are effective in dredging meridians, and improving local blood circulation.

4. Pressing and Kneading the Jianyu Point (LI 15)

Performance: Sitting position. The middle finger of one hand is used to press and knead Jianyu (located at the middle point above the deltoid muscle, between the acromion and greater tuberosity of humerus and in the depression anterior to the shoulder when the shoulder is raised up) on the affected side for about a minute until an aching and distending sensation is felt (see Fig. 5).

5. Pressing and Kneading the Jianliao Point (TE 14)

Performance: Sitting position. The middle finger of one hand is used to press and knead Jianliao (located in the depression below the posterior side of the prominence of acromion) (see Fig. 4) for about a minute until an aching and distending sensation is felt (see Fig. 6).

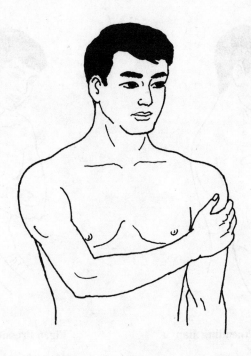

Fig. 3 Squeezing and kneading tenderness in the arm and shoulder

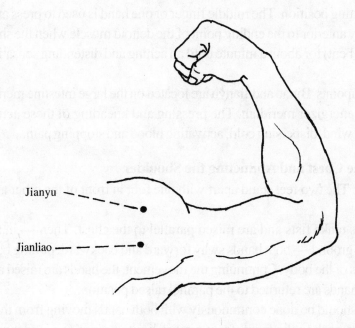

Fig. 4 Jianyu and Jianliao

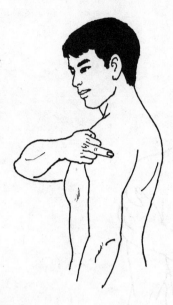

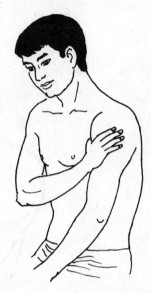

Fig. 5 Pressing and kneading Jianyu   **Fig. 6 Pressing and kneading Jianliao**

6. Pressing and Kneading the Binao Point (LI 14)

Performance: Sitting position. The middle finger of one hand is used to press and knead Binao (located slightly anterior to the ending point of the deltoid muscle when the shoulder is sunk and the elbow is bent) for about a minute until an aching and distending sensation is felt (see Fig. 8).

Among these acupoints, Binao and Jianyu are located on the large intestine meridian and Jianliao on the triple energizer meridian. The pressing and kneading of these acupoints is effective in dispelling wind, dispersing cold, activating blood and stopping pain.

7. Extending the Chest and Abducting the Shoulder

① Performance: The two feet stand apart with one foot in front of the other and knees slightly bent.

First, both hands make fists and are raised parallel to the chest. Then — in a rowing motion parallel to the ground — both hands sway forward and backward, pulling back as far as possible to the sides of the body. Continuing the movement, the hands are raised as high as possible. Finally the hands are returned to the parallel raised position.

These activities should be done continuously with both hands moving from the front to the back and from the back to the front, from a more limited range to a wider range like rowing a boat. This series of activities is done repeatedly for about a minute (see Fig. 9).

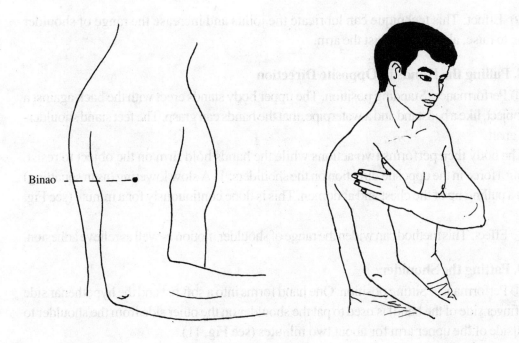

Binao - - - - - - - - - ●

Fig. 7 Binao   **Fig. 8 Pressing and kneading Binao**

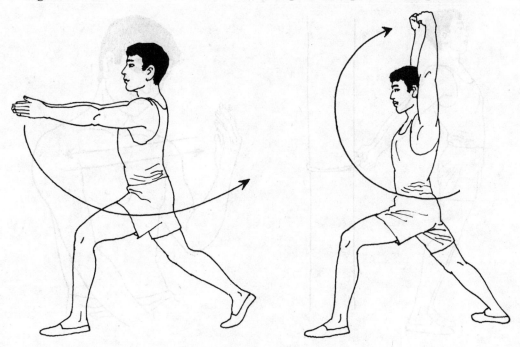

Fig. 9 Extending the chest and abducting the shoulders

② Effect: This technique can lubricate the joints and increase the range of shoulder motion to raise, abduct and twist the arm.

8. Pulling the Hands in Opposite Direction

① Performance: Standing position. The upper body stands erect with the back against a fixed object, like a bedstand and a waterpipe, that the hands can grasp. The feet stand shoulder-width apart.

The body then performs two actions while the hands hold firm on the object to resist, creating a force in the opposite direction on the shoulders: 1) A slow lowering (as in squatting) and 2) a pulling up of the chest and abdomen. This is done continuously for a minute (see Fig. 10).

② Effect: This method can widen the range of shoulder motion as well as relieve adhesion.

9. Patting the Shoulder

① Performance: Sitting position. One hand forms into a soft fist and the hypothenar side (little finger side of the hand) is used to pat the shoulder on the other side from the shoulder to the outside of the upper arm for about two minutes (see Fig. 11).

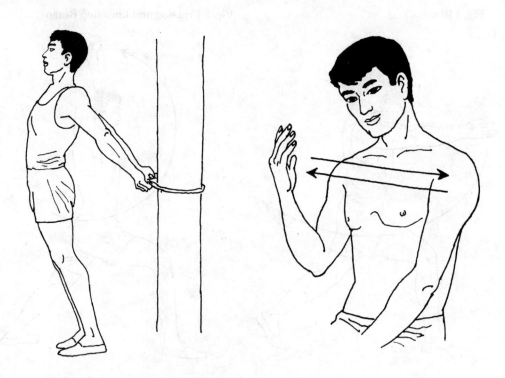

Fig. 10 Pulling the hands in opposite direction   **Fig. 11 Patting the shoulder**

② Effect: This method is effective in relaxing tendons, activating blood, warming and dredging meridians.

Notes:

1. Self-massage along meridians and acupoints is done one or two times a day according to the pathological conditions. This method is effective in reinforcing body resistance and preventing and treating scapulohumeral periarthritis.

2. Self-massage along meridians and acupoints should be done gently, slowly and gradually, avoiding any sudden movement.

3. Care should be taken to keep the shoulders warm and prevent cold and traumatic injury. In the evening, suitable clothing should be worn to keep the shoulders warm.

4. Clinical practice shows that scapulohumeral periarthritis tends to heal automatically. But the time it takes to heal can be very long, about one year. So timely treatment can shorten the healing process and alleviate pain.

Section 18 External Humeral Epicondylitis (Tennis Elbow)

Introduction

External humeral epicondylitis, also known as tennis elbow, is a common and widely encountered disease, usually seen among tennis and table tennis athletes, carpenters, fitters, water and electricity workers, middle-aged housewives and workers who wash and scrape floors. Currently it is generally believed that external humeral epicondylitis is caused by strain of the tendons through long-term and repeated stress on starting point of the muscle responsible for extending the wrist, resulting in chronic inflammation caused by lacerations of some muscular fibers. Other causes of humeral epicondylitis include retention of blood stasis due to local traumatic injury and obstruction of the meridians due to *qi* stagnation and blood stasis. Modern medical study shows that the causes of external humeral epicondylitis are various, such as the laceration of the general tendon of the forearm extensor, a local sprain, degenerative changes of the circular ligament of the radial head, periostitis of the external humeral epiphysis and bursal synovitis.

According to the pathogenesis of traditional Chinese medicine, the causes of external humeral epicondylitis are insufficiency of healthy *qi*, failure of blood to nourish the tendons and degenerative changes of the tendons. In the chapter of needling methods in *Suwen* (or *Plain Questions*), for example, it says that with sufficiency of healthy *qi* inside, pathogenic factors cannot attack the body. When the healthy *qi* is deficient and the defensive *qi* and myodynamia are weak, the body's ability to resist and adapt will be weakened. In this case, any slight traumatic injury may induce external humeral epicondylitis. Traumatic injury is, undoubtedly, an important factor responsible for this disease. The subjective symptoms of this disease are pain in the elbow, especially in the dorsiflexion of the wrist, bringing about much inconvenience for the patients in daily life and work.

The Symptoms of External Humeral Epicondylitis

In most cases the onset is slow, and the affected elbow experiences aching, distending, weakness and swelling. The pain is usually more severe at night and after work, often radiating to the forearm and wrist, middle and index fingers, or radiating to the upper arm and shoulder. In most cases, when forming a fist or rotating the hand (such as in twisting a towel), the pain worsens. In severe cases, the patient feels too weak to hold things or may drop things held in the hand.

In an examination, if there is tenderness in the external humeral condyle and if there is pain in the lateral part of the elbow whenever the elbow is stretched, the hand forms into a fist or the forearm turns in, the problem can be diagnosed as external humeral condylitis.

Self-Massage Along Meridians and Acupoints

1. Kneading the Arm on the Affected Side
① Performance: Sitting position. The elbow on the affected side is half bent and placed in front of the chest. The opposite hand then kneads it with all five fingers from the forearm to the lateral part of the upper arm and from the upper arm to the lateral part of the forearm for about five minutes (see Fig. 1).

② Effect: This technique can help relieve muscular tension on the affected side.

2. Pressing and Kneading Tenderness
① Performance: Sitting position. The elbow is placed on a table, palm down. The thumb of the opposite hand presses and kneads the external humeral condyle, especially the tender area. The massage should be gentle and slow at the start, gradually becoming stronger. This

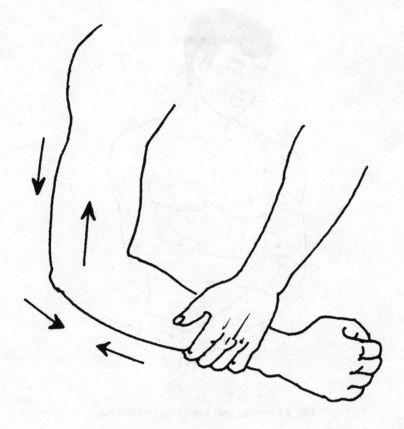

Fig. 1 Kneading the arm on the affected side

technique should be done repeatedly for about three minutes (see Fig. 2).

② Effect: This method can reduce stasis, disperse nodules and stop pain.

3. Pressing the Chize Point (LU 5)

Performance: Sitting position. The elbow on the affected side is half bent and the thumb of the opposite hand is used to press Chize (located on the transverse crease of the elbow and at the radial side of the tendon of brachial biceps) (see Fig. 3) for a minute until a local aching and distending sensation is felt (see Fig. 4).

4. Pressing the Shousanli Point (LI 10)

Performance: Sitting position. The elbow on the affected side is half bent and the thumb of the opposite hand is used to press Shousanli (located two *cun* below the ending point of

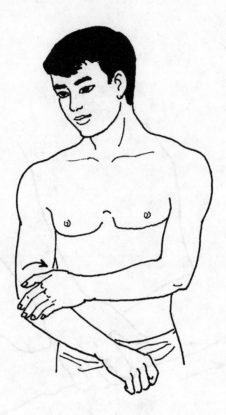

Fig. 2 Pressing and kneading tenderness

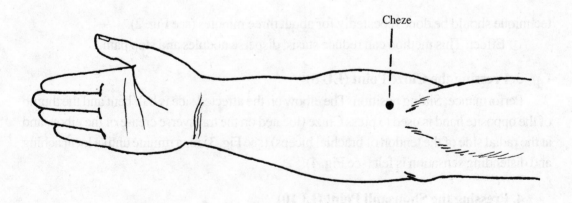

Fig. 3 Chize

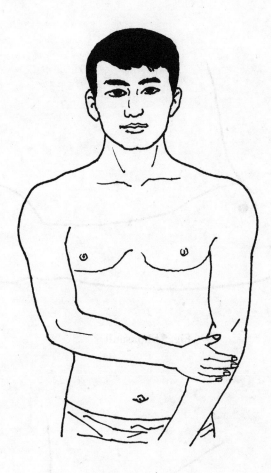

Fig. 4 Pressing Chize

the transverse crease of the elbow) for a minute until a local aching and distending sensation is radiated to the forearm (see Fig. 6).

Among the acupoints mentioned above, Chize is located on the lung meridian and Shousanli on the large intestine meridian. The pressing of these acupoints is effective in dredging meridians.

5. Stretching and Bending the Elbow

① Performance: Sitting position. The thumb on the healthy side presses the tender areas on the external humeral condyle and then the elbow is extended, bent or rotated repeatedly for about two minutes (see Fig. 7).

② Effect: This performance is effective in lubricating joints.

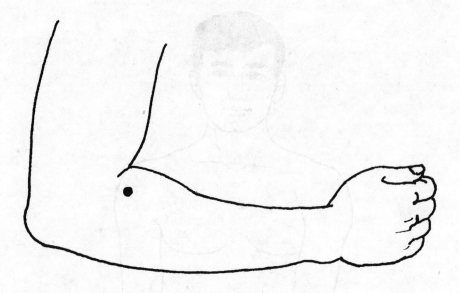

Fig. 5 Shousanli

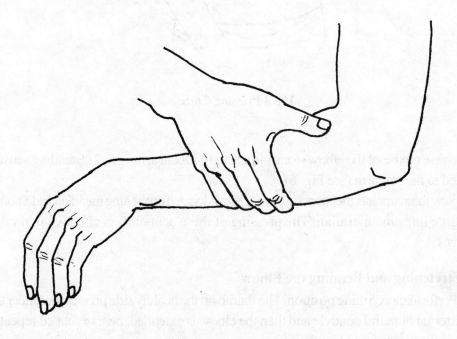

Fig. 6 Pressing Shoudanli

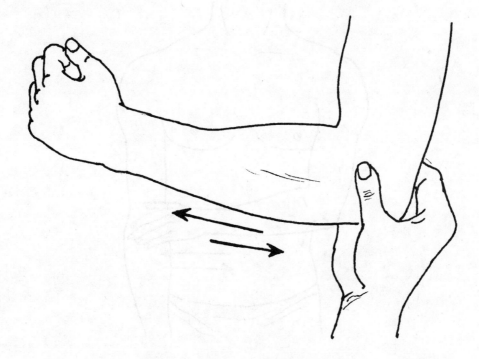

Fig. 7 Stretching and bending the elbow

6. Rubbing and Massaging the Elbow

① Performance: Standing or sitting position. The elbow on the affected side is stretched out, and the palm and fingers of the opposite hand — with the palm at the center — rub and massage along the outside of the elbow from the lower part of the upper arm to the upper part of the forearm for about two minutes until a local warm sensation is felt (see Fig. 8).

② Effect: This method can help warm and dredge meridians and promote local blood circulation.

Notes:

1. Self-massage along meridians and acupoints is done one or two times a day to dredge meridians, activate blood to disperse stagnation, relieve adhesion, smooth the circulation of *qi* and blood and warm muscles as well as moisten and nourish tendons and bones. In this way, the range of the motion in the elbow will be widened, the symptoms will be eliminated and the normal functions will be restored.

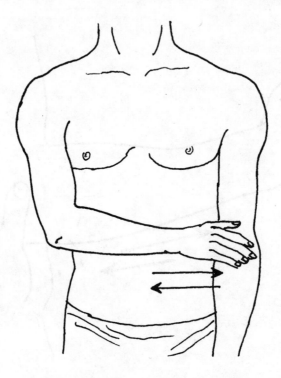

Fig. 8 Rubbing and massaging the elbow

2. A warm towel can be used as a compress on the affected part if there is swelling.

3. Take proper rest and avoid cold.

4. Care should be taken to reduce or discontinue movement of the elbow when there is pain.

5. Exercise can be done to move the elbow. But such activity should be moderate.

Section 19 Lumbar Muscle Strain

Introduction

Lumbar muscle strain is commonly encountered and is usually chronic and recurrent. It usually refers to a chronic injury of the soft tissues, such as lumbar muscles, fasciae, supraspinal ligament and sacro-iliac ligaments, etc.

This disease is usually caused by improper posture while working, or delayed or improper treatment after an acute lower back sprain, or sprain of the lumbosacral muscles and fascia due to repeated injury in the area of the waist or as a sequel to chronic lumbago. Sometimes lumbar muscle strain is caused by exposure to wind during sweating, lying in the open for cooling, attack by cold-dampness, overstrain and congenital deformity of the lumbosacral region.

Traditional Chinese medicine holds that the meridian over the waist pertains to *yang* and that the internal organ of the waist is the kidney and that the waist is the house of the kidney and that the various meridians pass through the waist. The meridian functions to transport *qi* and blood to nourish tendons and bones. Clinically, any impairment of the waist usually leads to damage of *qi* and blood inside and consequently results in stagnation of the meridians. Also, frequent invasion of wind-cold and dampness into the waist may lead to retention of pathogenic factors in the meridians and disharmony between *qi* and blood, eventually resulting in spasm and pain of the lumbar muscles and tendons.

The Symptoms of Lumbar Muscle Strain

The manifestation of this problem includes persistent chronic lumbago that reoccurs on one side or both sides of the waist. The problem may be light on one side and severe on the other. The pain is seldom sharp, usually manifesting as a distending pain, vague pain and ache. The symptoms may be aggravated after fatigue, but alleviated after rest. They become worse after a cold attack or on cloudy and rainy days. Usually the symptoms get alleviated during work or movement in the daytime, but return at night. In a few cases, aching pain appears in the buttocks and lateral upper part of the thigh. Examination reveals obvious tenderness at the region of strain and muscular tension or a rope-like hardness or nodules at the tender points.

Self-Massage Along Meridians and Acupoints

1. Pressing and Massaging the Lumbosacral Region

① Performance: Sitting position. Both hands form fists. The thumbs and the prominences of the metacarpophal-angeal articulation (thumb-side of the fist) are used to press and massage slowly and repeatedly from the waist to the sacrum for about five minutes (see Fig. 1).

② Effect: This method can help relax muscle spasms and relieve lumbosacral muscular lethargy.

2. Squeezing and Lifting the Lumbosacral Region

① Performance: Sitting position. The thumbs, index and middle fingers of both hands work to squeeze and lift the lumbar, back and sacral skin. Such massage is done lightly at first and then heavily from the upper to the lower for about two minutes (see Fig. 2).

② Effect: This method provides strong stimulation to relax tendons, activate collaterals and relax the lumbosacral muscles.

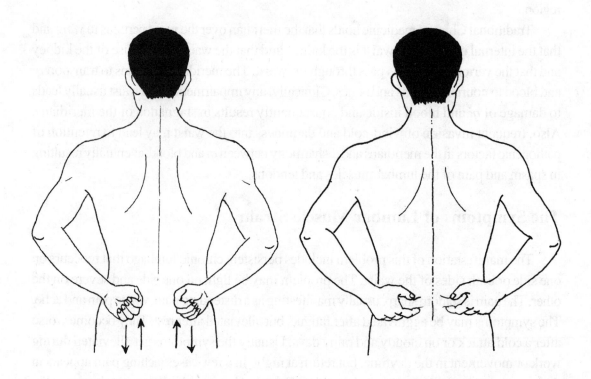

Fig. 1 Pressing and massaging the
lumbosacral region

Fig. 2 Squeezing and lifting the
lumbosacral region

3. Rotating the Waist

① Performance: Standing position. Both feet stand shoulder-width apart with both hands supporting the waist. With the waist taken as the axis, the upper body rotates slowly left, front, right and back for about half a minute; then rotates slowly from right, front, left and the back for half a minute (see Fig. 3).

② Effect: This method lubricates the lumbar joint.

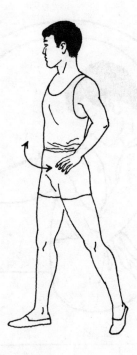

Fig. 3 Rotating the waist

4. Embracing the Knees to Bend and Stretch

Performance: Supination. Both hands embrace the knees, with the knees bent into the chest as close as possible. Then the legs stretch out and relax for a while. This is done repeatedly for about a minute (see Fig. 4).

5. Posterior Extension of the Arms and Legs

Performance: Prone position. Both legs are stretched out, and both hands are at the sides of the body. Then the head, chest and both arms and legs reach up and remain up for a while; then the head, chest and both arms and legs relax and rest for a while. This is done repeatedly for about a minute (see Fig. 5).

These two methods mentioned above are effective in regulating *qi* and blood as well as relaxing tendons and bones.

6. Stroking the Lumbosacral Region

Performance: Sitting position. The body leans slightly to the side at the waist. With open hands, fingers together, the hands are placed over the skin of the waist and back to stroke the lumbosacral region from the upper to the lower for about three minutes (see Fig. 6).

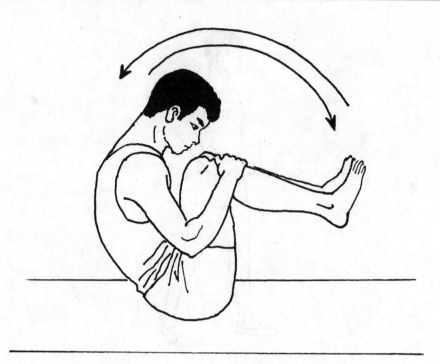

Fig. 4 Embracing knees to bend and stretch

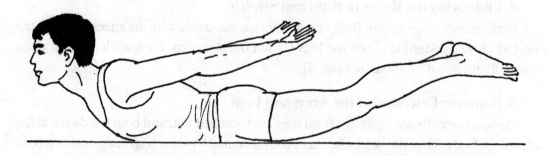

Fig. 5 Posterior extension of the arms and legs

7. Patting the Sacrum and the Buttocks

Performance: Standing position. The hands are formed into light fists that are used to pat the sacrum and the buttocks. The patting is done lightly and slowly at first and then heavily and swiftly. The massage is done repeatedly for about two minutes (see Fig. 7).

These two methods are effective in warming and dredging meridians, promoting the flow of *qi* and activating blood as well as expelling cold and relieving pain.

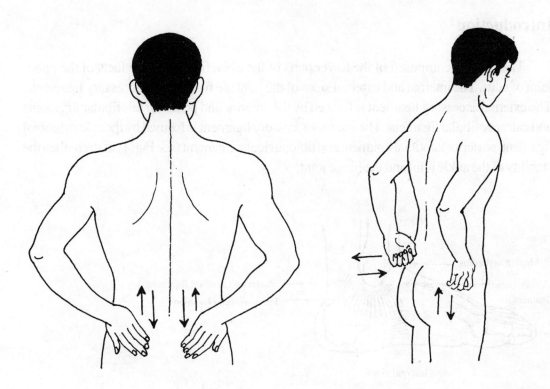

Fig. 6 Stroking the lumbosacral region   **Fig. 7 Patting the sacrum and the buttocks**

Notes:

1. Lumbar muscle strain is characterized by aching pain on one side or both sides of the lumbosacral region that is now light and then severe, lingering and recurrent. Therefore the patient should have confidence and do self-massage along meridians and acupoints one or two times a day. The massage increases blood circulation in the lumbosacral region, eliminates lumbar muscle overstrain, relieves lumbar muscular spasms, promotes the repair of strained muscles, ligaments and fasciae as well as strengthens the movement of the lumbosacral muscles, ligaments and fasciae.

2. It is advisable to use a wide belt to support the waist, sleep on a hard bed and frequently change posture and positions during working.

3. Keep the waist warm, reduce sexual activity and take care not to fall or do anything else that might cause lumbar sprain or bruising.

Section 20 Ankle Sprain

Introduction

The ankle is composed of the lower parts of the tibia, fibula and the facet of the upper joint of talus. The internal and external sides of the joint are fixed by the accessory ligaments. The external accessory ligament is formed by the anterior and posterior talofibular ligaments and calcaneofibular ligament. The internal accessory ligament is formed by the calcaneotibial ligament, posterior talotibial ligament and tibionavicular ligament (see Fig. 1) to strengthen the stability of the ankle joint and the hinge joint.

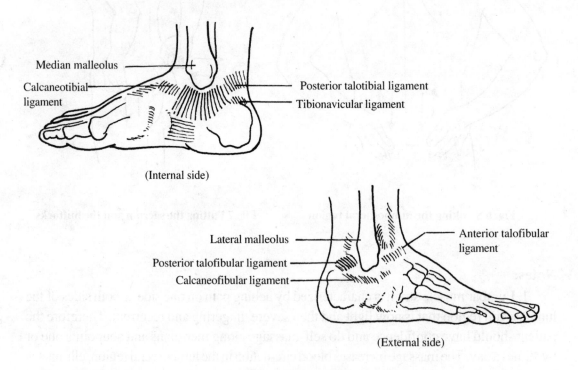

(Internal side)

(External side)

Fig. 1 Malleolus

Sprain of the ankle refers to any impairment of the soft tissues around the malleolus (the two rounded protuberances on each side of the ankle) due to sprain, excluding any fracture or dislocation of the malleolus. A sprained ankle may be caused by one foot slipping during walking, running, jumping, going downstairs and down a slope, which makes the body unstable due to the strong tensile force on the internal or external accessory ligament resulting from the excessive turning in or out of the malleolus, leading to a sprain. Clinically, the most common sprain occurs when an ankle twisted inward damages the accessory ligament of the lateral malleolus.

The Characteristics of the Symptoms of an Ankle Sprain

The main symptoms of an ankle sprain are pain, distension, limping or complete inability to walk, obvious tenderness over the affected part and a bluish discoloration of the skin in the affected region. If the lateral malleolus is sprained, the pain is obvious in the turning in of the foot. If the medial malleolus is sprained, the pain is obvious in the turning out of the foot, possibly accompanied by a laceration of the ligament. If both the medial and lateral malleoli are swollen and painful, careful examination must be done for an accurate diagnosis. X-ray examination should be taken if necessary.

Methods for Self-Massage Along Meridians and Acupoints

1. Pressing the Kunlun Point (BL 60)

Performance: Sitting position. The foot on the healthy side touches the ground with the knee bent. The thigh on the affected side is raised up and placed over the thigh of the healthy side.

The thumbs and index fingers are used to forcefully press Kunlun (located in the depression on the middle point of the line connecting the tip of the lateral malleolus and the Achilles tendon) on the affected side for one minute (see Fig. 2)

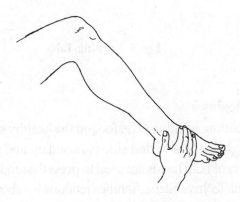

Fig. 2 Pressing Kunlun

2. Pressing the Taixi Point (KI 3)

Performance: Sitting position. The thumbs and index fingers are used to press Taixi (located on the middle point of the line connecting the tip of the medial malleolus and the Achilles tendon) on the affected side for about one minute (see Fig. 3).

Kunlun is located on the bladder meridian and Taixi on the kidney meridian. This method is effective in relaxing the tendons and dredging the collaterals.

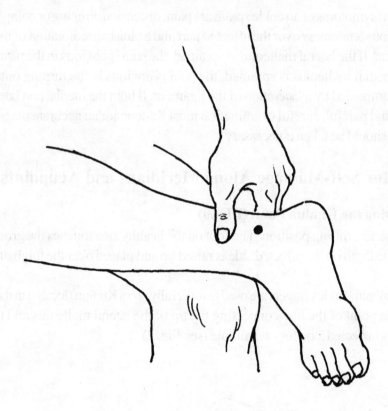

Fig. 3 Pressing Taixi

3. Pressing Malleolus

① Performance: Sitting position. The foot on the healthy side touches the ground with the knee bent. The thigh on the affected side is raised up and placed over the thigh at the healthy side. The fingers of both hands are used to press the tender area on the malleolus first and then to knead the malleolus and the Achilles tendons for about three minutes until pain in the affected part is alleviated (see Fig. 4).

② Effect: This method can reduce swelling and relieve pain.

4. Stroking Malleolus with the Foot

① Performance: Sitting position. The foot on the affected side touches the ground and the sole and heel of the foot on the healthy side touches the foot on the affected side and strokes forcefully from the upper to the lower. The sole of the foot on the healthy side is used to stroke the top of the foot on the affected side for a minute first. Then the sole and heel are used to scratch the medial malleolus for about a minute. Finally the top of the foot on the healthy side is crossed behind the heel of the affected side to stroke the lateral malleolus for about a minute. The stroking should be moderate and soft until a warm and comfortable sensation is felt in the affected part (see Fig. 5).

② Effect: This technique may warm and dredge meridians as well as reduce swelling and relieve pain.

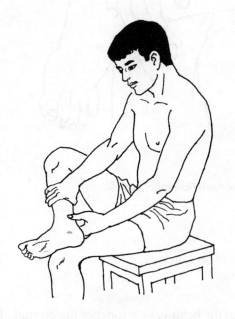
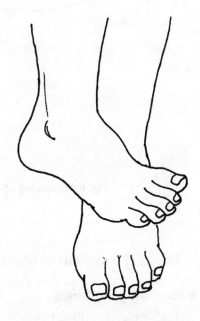

Fig. 4 Pressing malleolus   **Fig. 5 Stroking malleolus with the foot**

5. Squeezing and Holding the Gastrocnemius (calf) Muscle

① Performance: Sitting position. The foot on the healthy side touches the ground with knee bent. The thigh on the affected side is lifted and placed over the thigh on the healthy side. The fingers of both hands squeeze and hold the calf muscle from the back of the knee to the ankle for about two minutes. The massage should be even and soft, avoiding roughness (see Fig. 6).

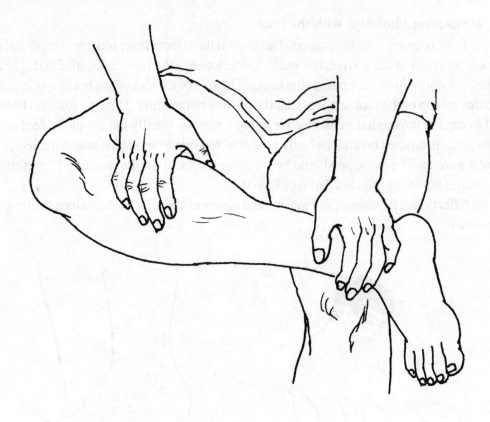

Fig. 6. Squeezing and holding the gastrocnemius muscle

② Effect: This method can help relax the meridians, and activates *qi* and blood.

6. Rounding the Ankle

① Performance: Sitting position. The foot on the healthy side touches the ground, the knee bent. The thigh on the affected side is lifted and placed over the thigh on the healthy side. One hand grasps the heel and the other hand grasps the sole to round to bend and pull the ankle lightly. The motion is done clockwise for half a minute and counterclockwise for half a minute from smaller to wider range (see Fig. 7).

② Effect: This method is effective in relaxing tendons, dredging collaterals and lubricating joints.

Notes:

1. Bone fracture or dislocation as well as torn tendons must be excluded before self-

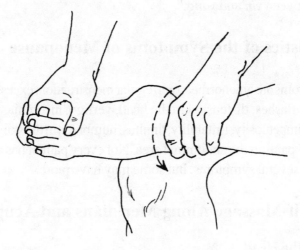

Fig. 7 Rounding the ankle

massage along meridians and acupoints can be applied.

2. Self-massage along meridians and acupoints should be done once a day. It is most effective in treating simple impairment of the malleolus ligament.

3. During the acute stage of an ankle sprain, care should be taken to walk less and rest more. The affected limb should be raised up while sleeping.

4. Care should be taken to prevent ankle sprains due to slipping when walking or jumping with a heavy load.

Section 21 Menopause

Introduction

At about the age of 50, the function of the ovary begins to decline in women and menstruation stops. At this time, disturbance of the nervous system and endocrine system may occur in some women before and after menopause, especially a disturbance of the autonomic nervous system.

According to traditional Chinese medicine, around the age of 50, menstruation stops due to "asthenia of the conception vessel, decline of the thoroughfare vessel, declination of kidney *qi* and imbalance between *yin* and *yang*."

The Characteristics of the Symptoms of Menopause

The usual symptoms are amenorrhea, or irregular menstruation, excessive flow or spotting accompanied by hot flashes, distension in the head, vertigo, insomnia, amnesia, sweating, palpitations, fatigue; impetuosity, irritability, tinnitus, numbness in the skin, or stabbing pain, or neuralgia and aching pains in the abdominal area. Not every patient has all these symptoms. Some may just have several symptoms, but some may have more.

Methods for Self-Massage Along Meridians and Acupoints

1. Percussing the Head
Performance: Sitting position. The fingers are slightly bent and separated. The tips of the fingers are used to percuss the head for about a minute (see Fig. 1).

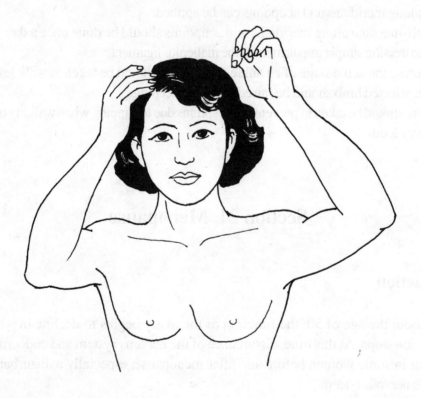

Fig. 1 Percussing the head

2. Stroking the Nape

Performance: Sitting position. The fingers of both hands intertwine and hold the nape with the head leaning slightly backward. Then both hands stroke and massage the nape forcefully for about two minutes (see Fig. 2).

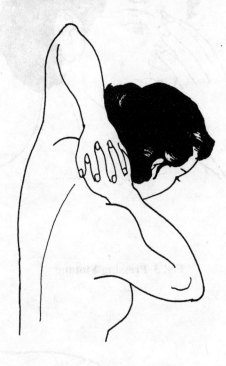

Fig. 2 Stroking the nape

These two methods are effective in refreshing the brain, and relieving vertigo, distension of head and headache.

3. Pressing the Yintang Point (EX-HN 3)

Performance: Sitting position. The middle finger of the right hand is used to press Yintang (located on the middle point of the line connecting the eyebrows) for about a minute (see Fig. 3).

4. Pressing the Neiguan Point (PC 6)

Performance: Sitting position. The thumbs of both hands are used to press Neiguan (located two *cun* directly above the middle point of the wrist crease and between the two tendons) at the opposite side for about a minute (see Fig. 4).

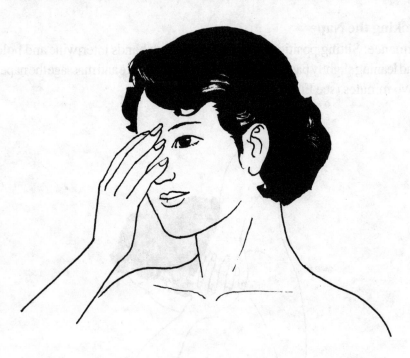

Fig. 3 Pressing Yintang

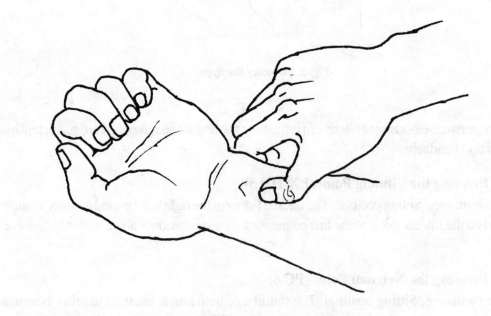

Fig. 4 Pressing Neiguan

5. Pressing the Xuehai Point (SP 10)

Performance: Sitting position. The thumbs of both hands are used to press Xuehai (located two *cun* directly above the medial and upper part of the patella) on the same side for about a minute (see Fig. 5).

6. Pressing the Sanyinjiao Point (SP 6)

Performance: Sitting position. The thumbs of both hands are used to press Sanyinjiao (located three *cun* directly above the medial malleolus tip and at the posterior border of the tibia) for about a minute (see Fig. 6).

Among these acupoints, Yintang is located on the extraordinary vessel, Neiguan on the pericardium meridian, and Sanyinjiao and Xuehai on the spleen meridian. The pressing of these acupoints is effective in dredging meridians and regulating *qi* and blood.

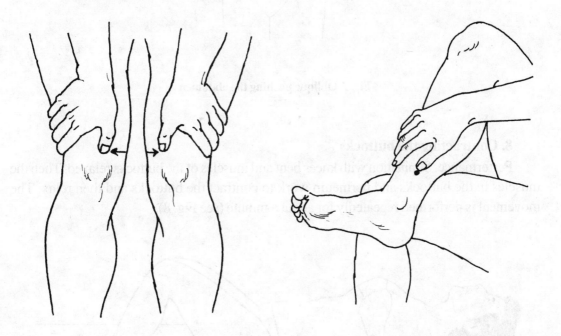

Fig. 5 Pressing Xuehai   Fig. 6 Pressing Sanyinjiao

7. Oblique Pushing of the Abdomen

Performance: Supination with the bending of the hips and knees and relaxation of the abdomen. The palms and fingers of both hands are placed on both sides of the abdomen to push into the abdomen down from the upper to the lower for about three minutes (see Fig. 7).

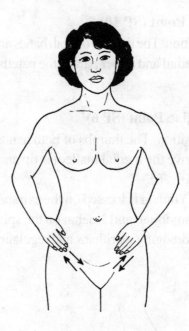

Fig. 7 Oblique pushing the abdomen

8. Contracting the buttocks

Performance: Supination with knees bent and muscles of the buttocks relaxed. Then the muscles in the buttocks and perineum work to contract the buttocks and then relax. The movement is performed repeatedly for about a minute (see Fig. 8).

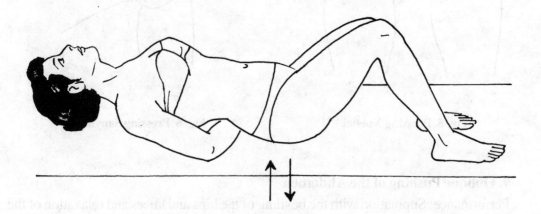

Fig. 8 Contracting the buttocks

These two methods are effective in promoting the flow of *qi*, activating blood, dispersing abdominal distension and relieving abdominal pain.

9. Pressing the Lumbosacral Region

① Performance: Sitting position with the head and chest leaning slightly backward. The palms and fingers of both hands are used to press the lumbosacral region from the upper to the lower for about three minutes (see Fig. 9).

② Effect: This method can help calm the mind.

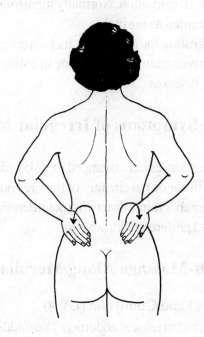

Fig. 9 Pressing the lumbosacral region

Notes:

1. Self-massage along meridians and acupoints is effective in treating and preventing symptoms associated with menopause. After being done one or two times a day continuously for 12 days, massage may be done once every other day according to the pathological conditions until the symptoms disappear. Usually symptoms are alleviated after three to five treatments. After 30 days of treatment, most patients are cured.

2. Patients should participate in proper physical exercise, pay attention to keeping a balance between work and rest and avoid mental stress.

Section 22 Irregular Menstruation

Introduction

Irregular menstruation refers to changes in the menstrual cycle as well as changes in the color, volume and texture of the blood. Actually, irregular menstruation includes early menstruation, delayed menstruation, unpredictable menstruation, excessive mensturation, scanty menstruation or an absence of menstruation. Normally menstruation occurs once a month. A few days earlier or later is regarded as normal.

The causes of irregular menstruation are various, including mental factors, excessive sexual activity, frequent childbirth, overstrain, intemperance in eating, attack by pathogenic cold, wind and dampness, or other diseases.

Characteristics of the Symptoms of Irregular Menstruation

The menstruation is irregular, either advanced or delayed. The menstruation is either profuse or scanty or spotty with abnormal changes of texture and color, usually accompanied by dizziness, aching back, lower abdominal distending pain, depression, irritability, palpitations, insomnia, aversion to cold and preference for warmth.

Manipulations for Self-Massage Along Meridians and Acupoints

1. Pressing Qihai (CV 6) and Guanyuan (CV 4)

Performance: Supination with a relaxed abdomen. The middle finger of one hand is placed on Qihai (located 1.5 *cun* below the navel) and Guanyan (located three *cun* below the navel) to press repeatedly into the abdomen for about a minute until a local aching and distending sensation is felt (see Fig. 1).

2. Pressing Daimai (GB 26)

Performance: Supination with the relaxation of the abdomen. The middle fingers of both hands are placed on Daimai (located directly below the free end of the eleventh rib and parallel to the navel) on both sides respectively and press repeatedly for about a minute (see Fig. 2).

3. Pressing Qichong (ST 30)

Performance: Supination. The thumbs of both hands are placed at Qichong (located five *cun* below Tianshu and at the femoral artery lateral and superior to the pubic tubercle) (see

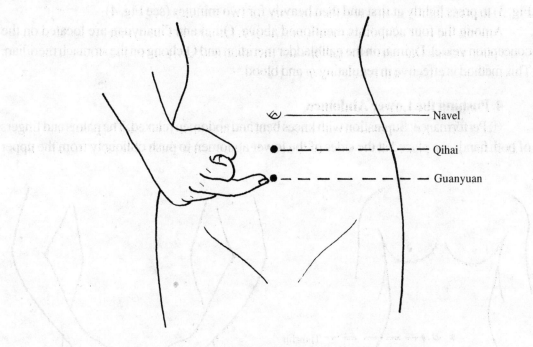

Navel

Qihai

Guanyuan

Fig. 1 Pressing Qihai and Guanyuan

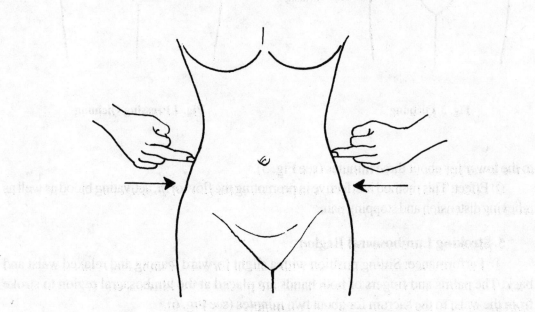

Fig. 2 Pressing Daimai

Fig. 3) to press lightly at first and then heavily for two minutes (see Fig. 4)

Among the four acupoints mentioned above, Qihai and Guanyuan are located on the conception vessel, Daimai on the gallbladder meridian and Qichong on the stomach meridian. This method is effective in regulating *qi* and blood.

4. Pushing the Lower Abdomen

① Performance: Supination with knees bent and abdomen relaxed. The palms and fingers of both hands are placed at the sides of the lower abdomen to push obliquely from the upper

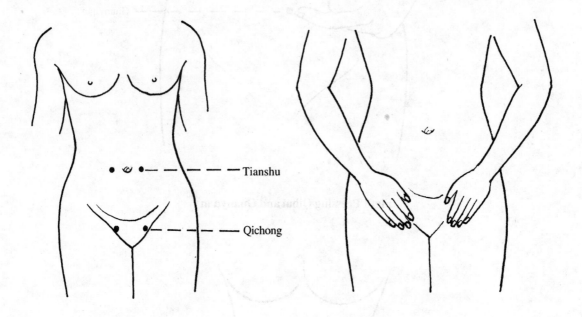

Fig. 3 Qichong	Fig. 4 Pressing Qichong

to the lower for about three minutes (see Fig. 5).

② Effect: This method is effective in promoting the flow of *qi*, activating blood as well as relieving distension and stopping pain.

5. Stroking Lumbosacral Region

① Performance: Sitting position with a slight forward leaning and relaxed waist and back. The palms and fingers of both hands are placed at the lumbosacral region to stroke from the waist to the sacrum for about two minutes (see Fig. 6).

② Effect: This method can help invigorate *qi* and nourish blood as well as warm meridians and disperse cold.

6. Percussing Baliao (the posterior sacral foramens)

① Performance: Sitting position. Both hands are formed into loose fists and the top sides of the fists are used to percuss the four posterior sacral foramens on both sides for about

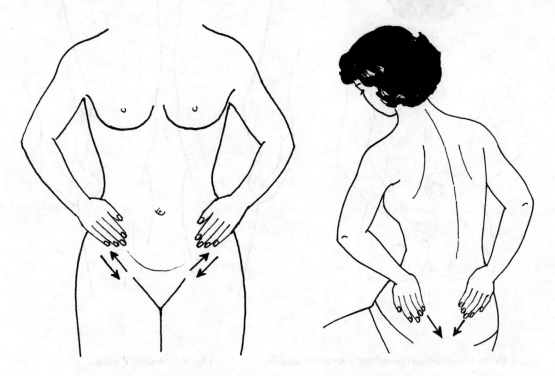

Fig. 5 Pushing the lower abdomen   **Fig. 6 Stroking the lumbosacral region**

two minutes (see Fig. 7).

② Effect: This technique can help invigorate *qi* and nourish blood as well as warm meridians and disperse cold.

7. Pressing Zusanli (ST 36)

Performance: Sitting position. The thumbs of both hands are used to press and pinch Zusanli (located three *cun* below Waixiyan and one transverse finger lateral to the tibia) at the same side for about two minutes until an aching and distending sensation radiates to the lower region (see Fig. 8).

8. Pressing Taichong (LR 3)

Performance: Sitting position. First the right foot is placed on the left leg, the right hand grasps the lower leg and the left thumb presses Taichong (located in the depression two *cun*

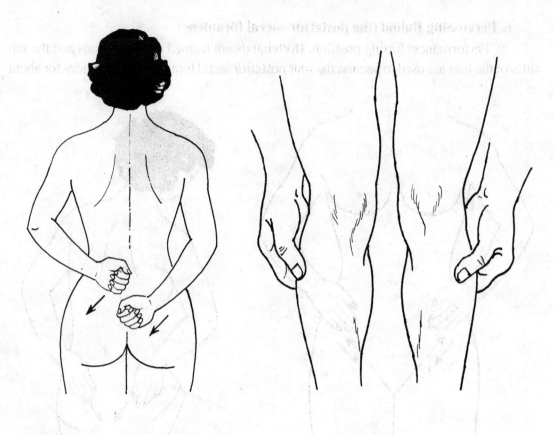

Fig. 7 Percussing Baliao (posterior sacral foramens)   **Fig. 8 Pressing Zusanli**

above the first and second digital fissures on the dorsum of the right foot) (see Fig. 9) for about a minute until an aching and distending sensation is felt (see Fig. 10). Then Taichong on the left foot is pressed in the same way.

Among these acupoints, Zusanli is located on the stomach meridian and Taichong on the liver meridian. The pressing of these acupoints is effective in regulating *qi*, nourishing blood and regulating menstruation.

Notes:

1. Self-massage along meridians and acupoints should be done one or two times a day and is discontinued during menstruation.

2. Pay attention to hygiene and keep the genitals clean during menstruation.

3. Daily life must be regular, avoiding overstrain and participating in appropriate physical exercises.

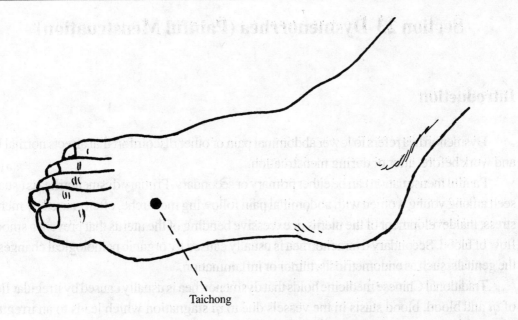

Fig. 9 Taichong

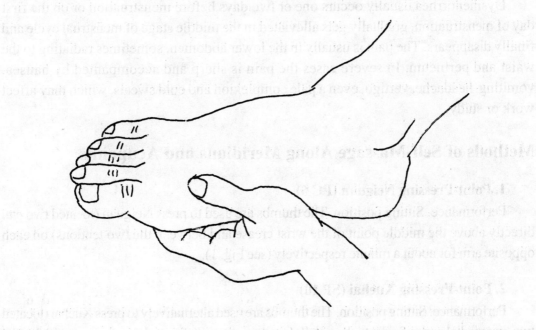

Fig. 10 Pressing Taichong

Section 23 Dysmenorrhea (Painful Menstruation)

Introduction

Dysmenorrhea refers to lower abdominal pain or other discomfort that affects normal life and work before, after or during menstruation.

Painful menstruation can be either primary or secondary. Primary dysmenorrhea is usually seen among young women with abdominal pain following menarche, often caused by mental stress, maldevelopment of the uterus or excessive bending of the uterus that prevent a smooth flow of blood. Secondary dysmenorrhea is usually caused by organic pathological changes of the genitals, such as endometriosis, tumor or inflammation.

Traditional Chinese medicine holds that dysmenorrhea is usually caused by irregular flow of *qi* and blood, blood stasis in the vessels due to *qi* stagnation which leads to an irregular menstrual flow and abdominal pain.

The Characteristics of the Symptoms of Dysmenorrhea

Dysmenorrhea usually occurs one or two days before menstruation or on the first day of menstruation, gradually gets alleviated in the middle stage of menstrual cycle and finally disappears. The pain is usually in the lower abdomen, sometimes radiating to the waist and perineum. In severe cases the pain is sharp and accompanied by nausea, vomiting, headache, vertigo, even a pale complexion and cold sweats, which may affect work or study.

Methods of Self-Massage Along Meridians and Acupoints

1. Point-Pressing Neiguan (PC 6)

Performance: Sitting position. The thumbs are used to press Neiguan (located two *cun* directly above the middle point of the wrist crease and between the two tendons) on each opposite arm for about a minute respectively (see Fig. 1).

2. Point-Pressing Xuehai (SP 10)

Performance: Sitting position. The thumbs are used alternatively to press Xuehai (located two *cun* medial and superior to the patella) on the same side for one minute respectively (see Fig. 2).

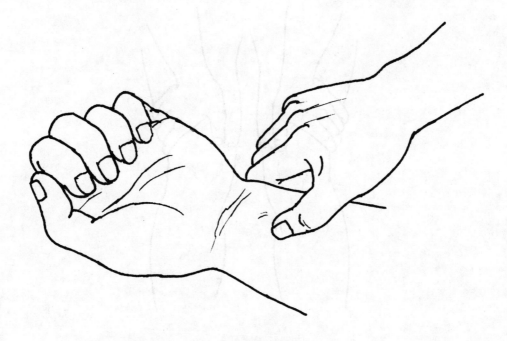

Fig. 1 Pressing Neiguan

3. Point-Pressing Sanyinjiao (SP 6)

Performance: Sitting position. The thumbs of both hands are used alternatively to press Sanyinjiao (located three *cun* directly above the tip of the medial malleolus and at the posterior border of the tibia) for one minute respectively (see Fig. 3).

4. Point-Pressing Gongsun (SP 4)

Performance: Sitting position. The thumb of one hand is used to press Gongsun (located at the anterior lower border of the first medial metatarsal bone base and at the red and white margin) (see Fig. 4) for about a minute until a local numb and distending sensation is felt (see Fig. 5). Then the other thumb is used to press Gongsun on the other foot in the same way.

Among the acupoints mentioned above, Neiguan is located on the pericardium meridian, Xuehai, Sanyinjiao and Gongsun on the spleen meridian. So this method is effective in dredging meridians and regulating *qi* and blood.

5. Pressing and Kneading the Abdomen

① Performance: Supination with knees bent and abdomen relaxed. The hands are placed

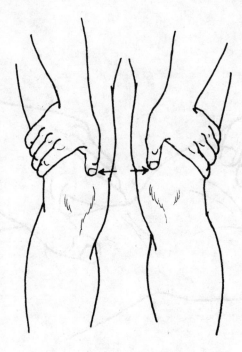

Fig. 2 Pressing Xuehai

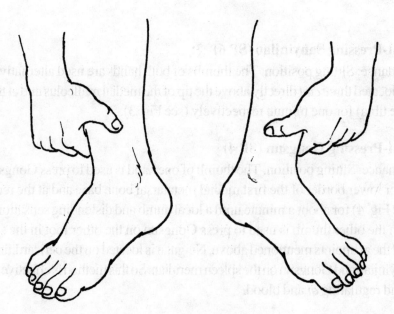

Fig. 3 Pressing Sanyinjiao

on top of each other to press and knead the abdomen with the navel to the center repeatedly, stirling clockwise from the right to the left for about five minutes until a local warm sensation is felt. The manipulation should be gentle and swift, light first and then heavy (see Fig. 6).

STEP 3: This method is effective in regulating qi and blood in the stomach and intestines.

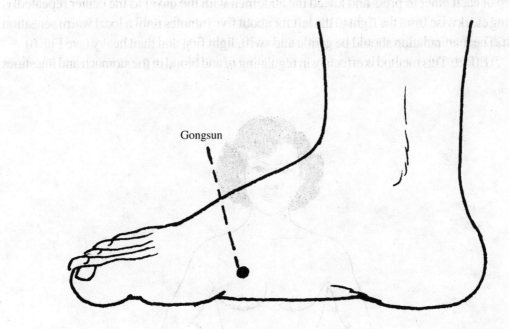

Fig. 4 Gongsun

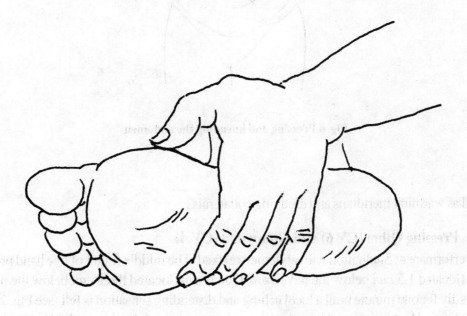

Fig. 5 Pressing Gongsun

on top of each other to press and knead the abdomen with the navel as the center repeatedly, starting clockwise from the right to the left for about five minutes until a local warm sensation is felt. The manipulation should be gentle and swift, light first and then heavy (see Fig. 6).

② Effect: This method is effective in regulating *qi* and blood in the stomach and intestines

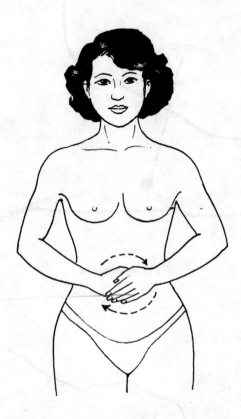

Fig. 6 Pressing and kneading the abdomen

as well as warming meridians and dredging collaterals.

6. Pressing Qihai (CV 6) and Guanyuan (CV 4)

Performance: Supination with abdomen relaxed. The middle finger of one hand presses Qihai (located 1.5 *cun* below the navel) and Guanyuan (located three *cun* below the navel) repeatedly for one minute until a local aching and distending sensation is felt (see Fig. 7).

Qihai and Guanyuan are located on the conception vessel. So this method is effective in regulating *qi* and blood and dredging meridians.

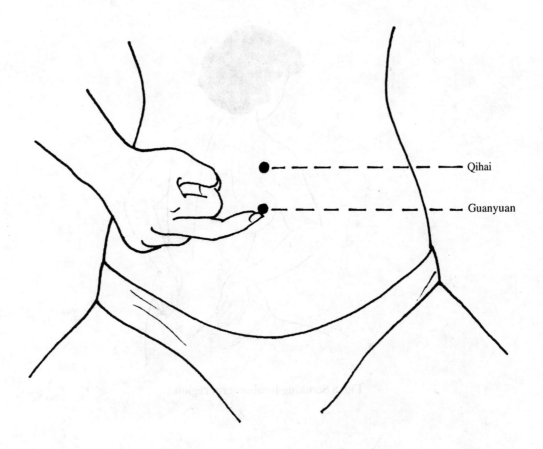

Qihai

Guanyuan

Fig. 7 Pressing Qihai and Guanyuan

7. Stroking the lumbosacral region

① Performance: Sitting position with the waist and back relaxed and bent slightly forward. The palms and fingers of both hands are placed at the lumbosacral skin to stroke from the waist to the sacrum for about two minutes (see Fig. 8).

② Effect: This technique can help invigorate *qi* and nourish blood as well as warm meridians and disperse cold.

8. Squeezing and holding the medial side of the thigh

① Performance: Sitting position with knees slightly bent.

The fingers of both hands are used alternatively to squeeze the inner thigh from the groin to the knee for about one minute (see Fig. 9).

② Effect: The inner thigh is the area through which the three *yin* meridians of the foot pass. So this method is effective in regulating meridian *qi* and relieving abdominal pain.

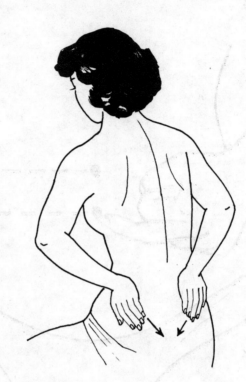

Fig. 8 Stroking lumbosacral region

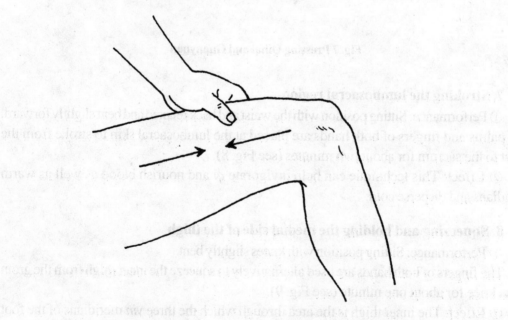

Fig. 9 Squeezing and holding the medial side of the thigh